PHARMACY:

An Introduction to the Profession

Readers

Recommended readings supplemental to this book will be posted annually on APhA's PharmacyLibrary (www.PharmacyLibrary.com).

PHARMACY:

An Introduction to the Profession
Third Edition

L. Michael Posey, BSPharm, MA
President
Pharmacy Editorial & News Services
Arlington, Virginia

Abir A. Kahaleh, BSPharm, MS, PhD, MPH
Associate Professor, Pharmacy Administration
Roosevelt University College of Pharmacy
Chicago, Illinois

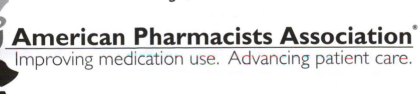

American Pharmacists Association®
Improving medication use. Advancing patient care.

APhA

Washington, D.C.

Acquiring Editor: Julian I. Graubart
Managing Editor: Meghan Reynolds
Copyeditors: Barbara Ann Bates and Linda Stringer, Publications Professionals LLC
Proofreader: Meghan Reynolds
Indexer: Mary Coe
Layout and Graphics: Michele A. Danoff, Graphics by Design
Cover Design: Julie Farrar, APhA Integrated Design and Production Center

© 2016 by the American Pharmacists Association
Published by the American Pharmacists Association
2215 Constitution Avenue, N.W.
Washington, DC 20037-2985
www.pharmacist.com   www.pharmacylibrary.com

This textbook was published from 1992 through 2002 as an annually updated serial titled *Pharmacy Cadence* by Pharmacy Editorial & News Services, Inc., Athens, Georgia.

To comment on this book via e-mail, send your message to the publisher at aphabooks@aphanet.org.

Library of Congress Cataloging-in-Publication Data

Names: Posey, L. Michael, author. | Kahaleh, Abir A., author. | American
  Pharmacists Association, issuing body.
Title: Pharmacy : an introduction to the profession / L. Michael Posey, Abir
  A. Kahaleh.
Description: Third edition. | Washington, DC : American Pharmacists
  Association, [2016] | Includes bibliographical references and index.
Identifiers: LCCN 2016032021 (print) | LCCN 2016032720 (ebook) | ISBN
  9781582122779 | ISBN 9781582122793 ()
Subjects: | MESH: Pharmacy | Pharmaceutical Services | Career Choice |
  Education, Pharmacy
Classification: LCC RS122.5 (print) | LCC RS122.5 (ebook) | NLM QV 21 | DDC
  615.1023–dc23
LC record available at https://lccn.loc.gov/2016032021

How to Order This Book

Online: www.pharmacist.com/shop
By phone: 800-878-0729 (from the United States and Canada)
VISA®, MasterCard®, and American Express® cards accepted

Dedication

To the pharmacists of tomorrow

Contents

Preface | to the Third Edition

As students pass through the years of undergraduate education in America's colleges of pharmacy, they are presented with the opinions and viewpoints of dozens of faculty members, the perspectives and outlooks of hundreds of journal articles and textbooks, and the intricacies of thousands—some would say millions—of facts. Sometimes, amid the cadence of all this information, the student never understands the bigger picture of how all the pieces fit together.

Since this textbook was first published in 2003, its purpose has been to provide a simple framework, in advance, so that students will know better what a certain term means or what an issue is all about. This updated third edition contains the latest information on the state of pharmacy today, including how patient care services now being provided by pharmacists are enhancing the practice of our profession.

During the doctorate of pharmacy program, the student is expected to undergo a process known as *professionalization*. This process can begin only when the student has developed an accurate view of the profession he or she is entering and has come to understand the basic tenets of the profession and the critical issues it is now facing.

Pharmacy: An Introduction to the Profession provides that basis for the budding pharmacy student. Written for orientation to pharmacy courses (at both the preprofessional and professional levels), this book has concise chapters focusing on the core knowledge needed to put information from other courses into perspective. The text is best supplemented with lectures from pharmacy faculty members or administrators with expertise in the various subject areas. Also, practitioners from various areas of pharmacy practice should be invited to supplement the discussion of pharmacy career paths (Chapter 6) and postgraduate education (Chapter 10). When colleges of pharmacy do not have a standalone orientation course, this text can be used for supplemental reading in an appropriate preprofessional—or early professional—level course.

Improvements in future editions of this textbook will be based on faculty and student feedback. Please contact us with ideas for expansion or improvement at the e-mail addresses shown below. Only through your input can this text gain more utility for tomorrow's students of pharmacy.

L. Michael Posey, BSPharm, MA (Lmposey@mac.com), Arlington, Va.

Abir (Abby) A. Kahaleh, BSPharm, MS, PhD, MPH (AKahaleh@roosevelt.edu), Chicago, Ill.

June 2016

Acknowledgments

Initial development of this book would not have been possible without the advice and suggestions of the pharmacy deans and faculty who were surveyed during planning stages. Bruce A. Berger of Auburn University contributed Chapter 4, "Communications in Pharmacy Practice," which summarizes concepts presented in his book *Communication Skills for Pharmacists,* 3rd edition, published by the American Pharmacists Association.

Chapter 1

Pharmacy's Cadence: Drumbeat of a Profession

L. Michael Posey and Abir A. (Abby) Kahaleh

Over the past 30 years, pharmacy has made a number of important decisions, ones that were very controversial among members of the profession. As we move toward the end of the second decade of the twenty-first century, we're happy to report to you that those difficult choices are reaping dividends for pharmacy and pharmacists.

As you will read in the pages of Chapters 2 and 3 of this textbook, the profession of pharmacy has a long and illustrious history, one filled with challenges that led pharmacists to adapt and innovate. In recent years, change required pharmacists to expand from a singular focus on the medication and an economic reliance on payments generated by the transfer of drugs and drug products to the patient. The profession, recognizing that new and more powerful medications were presenting challenges to physicians and patients alike, needed to expand from being a source of the medications to also providing patients with the information needed to safely and appropriately use those drugs.

Medication therapy management: Pharmacy's raison d'être

For centuries, pharmacists have been paid when they provided a medicinal agent or product to patients. This system served the profession well for millennia. When the responsibilities of medicine and pharmacy were demarcated a few centuries ago, pharmacists focused their practices on the art of preparing the medicinals prescribed by physicians using unique equipment available in their apothecaries and developed new ways of making medicinal agents palatable, effective, and safe.

Over a few decades in the late nineteenth and early twentieth centuries, the pharmaceutical industry gradually subsumed many of the compounding responsibilities of pharmacists, making the dispensing part of pharmacy not much more than counting and pouring from big bottles into little bottles, and then preparing a label and sticking it on the prescription vial or bottle. Pharmacy responded to this change in many ways, as is described more completely in Chapter 3. A key component of this response was to increase the medication information activities of pharmacists. For example, in some cases, pharmacists needed to contact physicians to suggest changes in prescriptions or even to decline to dispense a prescription that might harm the patient. The problem was that, in these cases, the pharmacist was not being reimbursed for the extra work, and if the prescription was not dispensed, no payment at all would occur.

The profession, starting in the 1960s and 1970s, developed information services, first in hospitals and then for patients in nursing homes. The systems were quickly incorporated into the institutional structures, and government regulations were soon developed for those settings. But patients in community pharmacies did not see much change. Because the public's overall perception of pharmacy relies on what they see in the com-

Learning Objectives

Upon completion of this chapter, the reader should be able to:

1. Highlight milestones in the profession of pharmacy.

2. Identify critical factors that led to the expansion of the role of pharmacists in public health.

3. Describe contemporary pharmacy practice models.

"Shallow men believe in luck, believe in circumstance. Strong men believe in cause and effect."

—Ralph Waldo Emerson

"Chance favors the prepared mind."

—Louis Pasteur

munity independent and chain pharmacy, people began to think that pharmacists really didn't do anything but "count, pour, lick, and stick."

Beginning with a federally mandated requirement to offer medication counseling to patients in the Medicaid program in the 1990s, this situation began to change in community pharmacies, but at a hopelessly glacial rate. As you will read in Chapter 3, the American Pharmacists Association (APhA) Foundation and motivated pharmacists in Asheville, North Carolina, finally created some movement in community pharmacies when they established and nurtured models for community pharmacists to use in providing a new kind of care to patients with chronic diseases such as diabetes and high serum cholesterol levels. The resulting practice, called *medication therapy management* (MTM),[1] was included in the 2003 legislation that created a prescription drug benefit for people with disabilities and senior citizens who receive health care under the federal Medicare program. In addition, pharmacists with the U.S. Army, working closely with APhA staff members, began to advocate that pharmacies were an ideal place for patients to be vaccinated against influenza and other infectious diseases. These events began to change the perception of the corner drugstore from a mercantile outlet to one where patients could obtain health care services.

Paradigm:
As used in this book, the typical or standard activities of a pharmacist on a day-to-day basis.

Pharmacy technician:
A paraprofessional assistant to the pharmacist who helps with the mechanical preparation of medications for dispensing to patients. This person may interpret prescription orders, prepare the medication (including some compounding of medications and preparation of intravenous solutions), and check the work of other technicians in specific situations.

The prospects for MTM making a tremendous difference are excellent. Independent pharmacies have implemented MTM programs, and some pharmacy chains have several pharmacists with special training in MTM in every unit. Pharmacy practitioners continue to work under an emerging **paradigm** that integrates accurate dispensing of the medications with MTM services that focus on how pharmacotherapy can improve the health of each patient.[2] Because the number of pharmacists is limited and the number of prescriptions dispensed annually is growing, accurate dispensing will rely on automation and **pharmacy technicians**, and pharmacies need to continuously develop sound systems for managing this process even as they meet with patients to discuss their use of medications.

An article in the APhA's MTM magazine, *Pharmacy Today*,[3] revealed that this mode of pharmacy practice works.[4-10] Employers whose budgets are being strained by health care costs ought to pay attention to the results afforded by pharmacist care of chronic diseases,[5,7,8] the model for pharmacist provision of such services has been tested and shown to work in a variety of pharmacy and geographic settings,[11] and pharmacists who have the knowledge, skills, and tools for delivering this type of care are available.[12,13]

With the 2010 passage of the of the Patient Protection and Affordable Care Act, better known as just the Affordable Care Act (ACA) or Obamacare, the role of pharmacists has expanded in the public health arena. In many ways, pharmacy previously had been an isolated profession. However, given increased concern over medication errors, decreased adherence to therapeutic regimens, unmet needs for primary care services, and availability of digital means for connecting geographically dispersed health settings, pharmacists are poised to practice at the top of their license.[14]

This chapter focuses on the importance of this legislation and its implications for pharmacy. It also covers other general trends to the profession: the need for the interprofessional team members to empower pharmacists in their expanding roles and the exploding demand for medications and health care in general because of the number of senior citizens in the United States and other developed countries. Pharmacists and future practitioners need the information, support, resources, and opportunity to provide efficient and high-quality transition of care in various practice settings.[15,16]

Accountable care organizations

One of the contemporary models of pharmacy practice is the accountable care organization (ACO). ACOs are being established as the ACA is implemented. The ACO model was developed as an alternative payment mechanism to decrease the rising costs of the fee-for-service approach and to enhance the quality of care.[17] Under the model, a network of practitioners and hospitals provide health care services to patient populations.[18] The group is responsible for the financial and clinical outcomes of patients. Pharmacists play a vital role in providing MTM and in collaborating with a team of interprofessional clinicians.

Patient-centered medical homes

Another effective approach to providing efficient and high-quality services is the patient-centered medical home (PCMH). In the PCMH model, pharmacists provide care using a team approach. The successful development, integration, and sustainability of having a pharmacist in the PCMH depend on the recognition of their critical role as the medication experts.

Several recent publications have highlighted the vital role of pharmacists in PCMHs. A study from North Carolina examined the contributions of pharmacists during the transition of care and in ambulatory care settings.[19] The researchers concluded that pharmacists and student pharmacists effectively provided needed direct patient care services and interprofessional education in pharmacotherapy, anticoagulation, and osteoporosis clinics.

Likewise, a study of Blue Cross Blue Shield of Michigan examined the effects of having pharmacists in PCMHs.[20] The researchers evaluated pharmacists' direct patient care services in eight general medicine health centers. The patients at the centers suffered from chronic diseases, including diabetes, hypertension, and hyperlipidemia. Results of the study showed that the PCMH pharmacists provided direct patient care an average of 2.2 days per week in various clinics. Specifically, the pharmacists reviewed the patients' medications and made recommendations for medication changes for patients with diabetes and provided consultations on hypertension, hyperlipidemia, and polypharmacy.

Pharmacists in public health

With the increasing emphases on population health and preventive care, the role of pharmacists in public health is expected to continue to expand. When this text was revised in mid-2016, the number of pharmacy students was approaching 65,000 and the number of colleges and schools of pharmacy was 135. Current and future pharmacists are poised to enhance population health.[21]

Several initiatives have been undertaken to address population health, including the Healthy People initiative. This macro-level initiative has guided public health work in the United States for the past three decades.[22]

As the most accessible health care professionals, pharmacists can provide care to the medically underserved patient populations.[23] Furthermore, they can play a vital role in prevention and management of chronic diseases by integrating behavioral health and implementing frameworks for health promotion and education programs among the aging patient population.[24]

Health care: Economics of aging for the baby boomers

The world is changing. As a result of advances in medical science, people are living longer, especially in developed countries but also in developing countries. Combined with a decreasing birth rate in many countries, the world's population is becoming older. As shown in Figure 1.1, the number of people in the retired age groups is predicted to be far larger than it has been in the past, both in numbers and as a percentage of the population. All in all, the percentage of Americans who are 65 years of age or older will increase from 12.4% in 2000 to 19.6% in 2030.[25-27] Older people have more diseases—especially degenerative conditions such as arthritis and Alzheimer's disease—that interfere with their ability to walk, bathe, dress, feed themselves, or use the bathroom without assistance. Older patients generally also take many more medications than do younger people.

The implications of this demographic shift are far reaching. In the United States, millions of older Americans rely on the Social Security and Medicare programs for basic social and medical care. These programs depend on continued contributions from current workers to pay benefits for recipients, and the number of workers per retired person is falling. As the 76 million baby boomers—those Americans born between 1946 and 1964—are now

Figure 1.1 | **Critical job factors for pharmacy careers. Use this chart to ask yourself what you feel is important in your future pharmacy career.**

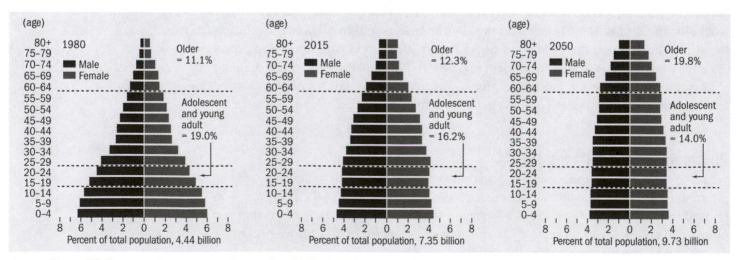

Source: Bloom DE. Demographic upheaval. Finance Dev. 2016;53(1): 6–11, chart 3.

reaching retirement age, the existing system for social and health care of senior citizens is increasingly stressed. Combine that fact with America's already burgeoning national debt, and the question of how America will pay for care of its senior citizens in the coming half-century becomes even more challenging. Can fewer and fewer workers pay enough in taxes to provide support for an increasing number of senior citizens and service the national debt at the same time? If not, what then?

For pharmacists, will these changes translate into a population whose chronic diseases are a natural fit for the kind of MTM services described in this chapter? Or will the continually increasing cost of medications simply mean that fewer and fewer resources are left over to pay for the professional expertise needed to use those medications properly?

Although no one knows the answers to such questions, the indicators for pharmacy are positive. First, drug-related problems (DRPs) are undoubtedly one of the big challenges facing the medical system in general and pharmacists in particular. Studies that are now nearly 20 years old showed that the annual cost of DRPs among ambulatory Americans (not counting those in hospitals and nursing homes) was $177 billion. For every $1 spent on medications, another $1 is spent paying for problems associated with use of the medications.[28] Experts who have analyzed DRPs conclude that, although a lot of DRPs are unexpected and cannot be foreseen, pharmacists could have prevented or minimized many DRPs through timely interventions.

In addition to pharmacists' receiving payment for such services under the Medicare Part D MTM program, the possibility that patients might pay pharmacists directly for help with managing medications is a positive sign.[29,30] As a sufficient number of patients experience MTM services and conclude that they are valuable, a tipping point may be reached that will lead to widespread patient demand for pharmacists' services. If and when that occurs, coverage by **pharmacy benefits managers** and other third-party payers will be common.

> **Pharmacy benefits managers (PBMs):**
> Companies that contract with managed-care organizations, insurance companies, or employers to provide prescriptions and pharmaceutical care to a covered population. PBMs often contract with networks of independent or chain pharmacies to provide this care in accordance with guidelines and rules that can reduce the cost of prescriptions.

If pharmacists are preoccupied with detecting and preventing DRPs, who will be responsible for getting the right drug to the right patient at the right time? Fortunately, several trends have converged to provide pharmacists with a lot of assistance in the process of drug preparation.

Pharmacists getting out of drug preparation

Pharmacists have for years had helpers who assisted with various tasks in the pharmacy and have used tools to make the job easier or faster. Advances in technology are producing sophisticated dispensing machines and robotic devices that, using bar code scanners, are virtually replacing pharmacists in their dispensing roles. Likewise, pharmacy technicians have emerged as an identifiable group of competent assistants who can perform many of the tasks formerly handled by pharmacists.

As applied in pharmacy practice, automated devices include systems for dispensing tablets and capsules. These systems generally combine a computer, a bar code scanner, and a counting device. Some systems produce strip packs of medications sealed into individual pouches; others put all the medications for a certain time of administration into a single pouch.

Automated dispensing systems are now being linked to computerized physician order entry systems in both hospitals and ambulatory settings. Medication errors caused by poor handwriting and other types of ineffective communication are driving physicians to write prescriptions on computers and personal digital assistants,[31] and Medicare Part D is expected to mandate an increased level of computerized physician order entry.

Robotic devices are more common in hospitals. Some robots deliver medications to nursing stations located around the building, whereas others are used to fill patient cassettes in unit-dose dispensing systems.[32]

Many exciting changes have been made with respect to the training, recognition, and legal status of pharmacy technicians. These paraprofessionals assist with the process of filling prescriptions. Although the tasks that technicians may legally perform vary from state to state, they generally include reading the physician's order, entering the information into a computer, placing the drugs into a container for the patient, affixing the label, and giving the completed materials to a pharmacist for checking.

Pharmacies that rely on technicians heavily—such as chain pharmacies, mail-service operations, and hospitals—often have formal training programs that combine classroom work with on-the-job experience. Additionally, community colleges and technical schools are implementing more and more training programs for technicians. The programs usually require one or two years of schooling. The U.S. military has an excellent training program for technicians.

In response to the advancing level of importance of pharmacy technicians within the practice, a national certification examination was established for pharmacy technicians. Housed physically within the headquarters of the American Pharmacists Association, the Pharmacy Technician Certification Board is an independent organization responsible for administering the examination, which tests the knowledge of pharmacy technicians. First administered in 1995, the examination has a high rate of passage—usually above 80%. The number of certified pharmacy technicians (CPhTs) exceeded 550,000 by 2015. Currently, the number of licensed pharmacists in the United States is about 290,000.[33] More information regarding pharmacy technician accreditation regulations, standards, processes, and procedures can be found at www.ashp.org/accreditation-technician.

Planning for change

As the quotations at the beginning of this chapter indicate, pharmacy has two choices in dealing with the breakneck pattern of change sweeping through health care: plan and prepare for it, or hope for the best. On the assumption than the former option is preferred, *Pharmacy: An Introduction to the Profession* will present the history, forces, trends, and concepts that influence pharmacy in its present state. You—the new student pharmacist in the early decades of a new millennium—can use this information in planning for the future of your new profession, pharmacy.

REFERENCES

1. American Pharmacists Association and National Association of Chain Drug Stores Foundation. Medication therapy management in pharmacy practice: core elements of an MTM service model (version 2.0). *J Am Pharm Assoc.* 2008;48(3):341-53.
2. Posey LM. Proving that pharmaceutical care makes a difference in community pharmacy [editorial]. *J Am Pharm Assoc.* 2003;43(2): 136-9.
3. Posey LM. MTM: the pieces fit together. *Pharm Today.* 2008:14(3).
4. Cranor CW, Christensen DB. The Asheville Project: short-term outcomes of a community pharmacy diabetes care program. *J Am Pharm Assoc.* 2003;43(2):149-59.
5. Cranor CW, Bunting BA, Christensen DB. The Asheville Project: long-term clinical and economic outcomes in a community pharmacy diabetes care program. *J Am Pharm Assoc.* 2003;43(2):173-84.
6. Garrett DG, Martin LA. The Asheville Project: participants' perceptions of factors contributing to the success of a patient self-management program for diabetes. *J Am Pharm Assoc.* 2003;43(2):185-90.
7. Bunting BA, Cranor CW. The Asheville Project: long-term clinical, humanistic, and economic outcomes of a community-based medication therapy management program for asthma. *J Am Pharm Assoc.* 2006;46(2):133-47.
8. Bunting BA, Smith BH, Sutherland SE. The Asheville Project: clinical and economic outcomes of a community-based long-term medication therapy management program for hypertension and dyslipidemia. *J Am Pharm Assoc.* 2008;48(1):23-31.
9. Bluml BM, McKenney JM, Cziraky MJ. Pharmaceutical care services and results in Project ImPACT: Hyperlipidemia. *J Am Pharm Assoc.* 2000;40(2):157-65.
10. Bluml BM, Garrett DG. Patient self-management program for diabetes: first-year clinical, humanistic, and economic outcomes. *J Am Pharm Assoc.* 2005;45(2):130-7.
11. Fera T, Bluml BM, Ellis WM, et al. The Diabetes Ten City Challenge: interim clinical and humanistic outcomes of a multisite community pharmacy diabetes care program. *J Am Pharm Assoc.* 2008;48(2):181-90.
12. Schommer JC, Planas LG, Johnson KA, Doucette WR. Pharmacist-provided medication therapy management (part 1): provider perspectives in 2007. *J Am Pharm Assoc.* 2008;48(3):354-63.
13. Schommer JC, Planas LG, Johnson KA, Doucette WR. Pharmacist-provided medication therapy management (part 2): payer perspectives in 2007. *J Am Pharm Assoc.* 2008;48(4):478-86.
14. Anderson S. Community pharmacy and public health in Great Britain, 1936 to 2006: how a phoenix rose from the ashes. *J Epidemiol Community Health.* 2007;61(10):844-8.
15. Kahaleh AA, Gaither C. The effects of work setting on pharmacists' empowerment and organizational behaviors. *Res Social Adm Pharm.* 2007;3(2):199-222.
16. Kahaleh AA, Cook GR. Pharmacy students providing medication discharge counseling. *US Pharm.* 2009;34(8):49-57.
17. Amara S, Adamson RT, Lew I, Slonim A. Accountable care organizations: impact on pharmacy. *Hosp Pharm.* 2014;49(3):253-9.
18. Colla CH, Lewis VA, Beaulieu-Jones BR, Morden NE. Role of pharmacy services in accountable care organizations. *J Manag Care Spec Pharm.* 2015;21(4):338-44.
19. Scott MA, Hitch B, Ray L, Colvin G. Integration of pharmacists into a patient-centered medical home. *J Am Pharm Assoc.* 2011;51(2):161-6.
20. Mi Choe H, Farris KB, Stevenson JG. Patient-centered medical home: developing, expanding, and sustaining a role for pharmacists. *Am J Health-Syst Pharm.* 2012:69(12):1063-71.
21. The role of the pharmacist in public health. American Public Health Association website. www.apha.org/policies-and-advocacy/public-health-policy-statements/policy-database/2014/07/07/13/05/the-role-of-the-pharmacist-in-public-health. Accessed May 12, 2016.
22. U.S. Department of Health and Human Services Office of Disease Prevention and Health Promotion. Healthy People 2020 website. www.healthypeople.gov. Accessed May 12, 2016.
23. Murphy PA, Frazee SG, Cantlin JP, Cohen E, Rosan JR, Harshburger DE. Pharmacy provision of influenza vaccinations in medically underserved communities. *J Am Pharm Assoc.* 2012;52(1):67-70.
24. Kahaleh AA, Youmans SL, Bresette JL, Truong HA. Health behavior theories and models: frameworks for health promotion and health education programs. In: Truong H-A, Bresette JL, Sellers JA, eds. *The Pharmacist in Public Health: Education, Applications, and Opportunities.* Washington, D.C.: American Pharmacists Association; 2010:159-80.

25. Institute of Medicine. *Retooling for an Aging America: Building the Health Care Workforce*. Washington, D.C.: National Academies Press; 2008.

26. Centers for Disease Control and Prevention. Public health and aging: trends in aging—United States and worldwide. *Morb Mortal Wkly Rep*. 2003;52(6):101–6.

27. Posey LM. America ages, pharmacy prepares. *Pharm Today*. 2003;9(5):1,11,13.

28. Ernst FR, Grizzle AJ. Drug-related morbidity and mortality: updating the cost-of-illness model. *J Am Pharm Assoc*. 2001;41(2):156–7.

29. Ganther JM. Third party reimbursement for pharmacist services: why has it been so difficult to obtain and is it really the answer for pharmacy? *J Am Pharm Assoc*. 2002;42(6):875–9.

30. Winckler SC. Pharmacist services: insurance need not be the only answer [editorial]. *J Am Pharm Assoc*. 2002;42(6):826.

31. Posey LM. Electronic physician order entry: segue to a fully automated medication system. *Pharm Today*. 2001;7(9):1,9,10.

32. Posey LM. Medication errors: the pain, the problems, the process. *Pharm Today*. 2001;7(2):1,21.

33. Occupational employment statistics. U.S. Bureau of Labor Statistics website. www.bls.gov/oes/current/oes291051.htm#nat. Updated March 30, 2016. Accessed May 12, 2016.

Chapter 2 | Development of Pharmacy in History as a Healing Profession

L. Michael Posey

For as long as the human species has encountered disease, injury, and illness, people have sought relief. Several detailed accounts of pharmacy history are available for the interested reader[1-3]; presented here is a brief overview of the roots of this profession. Noteworthy are the 40 original oil paintings commissioned by Parke–Davis, now a part of Pfizer, and recently donated to the American Pharmacists Association (APhA).[3] The development of this Robert Thom series—which is available online at www.pharmacist.com[4]—has been reviewed by George Griffenhagen, APhA's long-serving historian.[5] Reproductions of this series hang in many schools of pharmacy across the United States. Griffenhagen has also compiled the history of pharmacy as recorded on stamps and postal imprints.[6] An excellent illustrated history of pharmacy has been published, written by respected historians David L. Cowen and William H. Helfland.[7] Tables 2.1 through 2.6 provide interested students with detailed listings of key dates in pharmacy and world history.

In this chapter, we will study the history of pharmacy from its origins in ancient Babylonia through the middle of the twentieth century, when pharmacy's status as a profession was questioned by medicine and other parts of society. Chapter 3 details the more recent history of pharmacy as a process of reprofessionalization took hold.

Pharmacy in ancient times

Pharmacy was undoubtedly "practiced" in prehistoric times as people instinctively used the water, plants, and earth around them for soothing compresses on wounds and ailments. As civilization dawned in ancient Mesopotamia (2600 B.C.), Babylonian healing practitioners combined the responsibilities of priest, physician, and pharmacist,[3] and some of the oldest pharmacy records are found in Sumerian (Babylonian) clay cuneiform tablets that date to about 2000 B.C. Retailers of drugs were concentrated on a certain street in Babylon by 2111 B.C.[1,3,8]

In ancient China (circa 2000 B.C.), legend tells that Emperor Shen Nung investigated the medicinal properties of hundreds of herbs, and he recorded 365 native herbal drugs in the first Pen T'sao.[3]

Egyptian priests, as part of their duties, prepared medicines. The Ebers papyrus, which dates from 1900 to 1100 B.C., is the best-known and most important pharmaceutical record from ancient history. It contains 800 prescriptions using 700 drugs. Of particular note in the papyrus is inclusion of quantities of substances, which were largely missing in the Babylonian clay tablets. Many modern dosage forms are also referred to in the Ebers papyrus—gargles, snuffs, inhalations, suppositories, fumigations, enemas, poultices, decoctions, infusions, pills, troches, lotions, ointments, and plasters.[1]

Learning Objectives

Upon completion of this chapter, the reader should be able to:

1. Outline the history of pharmacy from prehistoric times to the middle of the twentieth century.

2. Recognize important world events as they relate to the development of pharmacy and medicine as professions.

3. Recognize important leaders who contributed to the development of pharmacy as a healing profession.

"... if the preparation of medicines is taken from the apothecary and he becomes merely the dispenser of them, his business is shorn of half its dignity and importance, and he relapses into a simple shopkeeper."

—William Procter, 1858

Table 2.1 | Selected World & Pharmacy Events Before the Middle Ages

Year	Event	Year	Event
50,000 B.C	Neanderthal man existed on Earth.	429–347 B.C.	Plato.
35,000 B.C.	Cro-Magnon man existed (late Paleolithic Age).	384–322 B.C.	Aristotle.
7000–2000 B.C.	Neolithic Age in Europe.	338–323 B.C.	Alexander the Great.
5000–4500 B.C.	Dawn of Sumerian, Egyptian, and Minoan cultures.	44 B.C.	Julius Caesar assassinated.
2500 B.C.	Surgical operations depicted in Egyptian pyramids.	4 B.C.	Jesus Christ born.
2000–1000 B.C.	Bronze Age in Europe.	79	Plague following eruption of Vesuvius. Pompeii destroyed.
1500 B.C.	Ebers papyrus.	130–201	Galen.
1237 B.C.	Death of Asclepius.	220	Han Dynasty ended in China.
1000–500 B.C.	Earlier Iron Age in Europe.	303	Martyrdom of Saints Cosmas and Damian (patron saints of medicine and pharmacy).
950 B.C.	Homer.	369	Hospital of St. Basil erected at Caesarea by Justinian.
753 B.C.	Founding of Rome.	395–1453	Byzantine Empire.
600 B.C.	Massage and acupuncture practiced by Japanese.	400	First hospital established in Western Europe.
580–489 B.C.	Pythagoras.	476	Fall of Roman Empire.
550 B.C.	Buddha and Confucius lived.		
525 B.C.	Asclepius raised to rank of God of Medicine in Greece.		
522 B.C.	Medical school founded at Athens.		
500 B.C.	Later Iron Age.		
460–361 B.C.	Hippocrates.		

Source: Adapted from Bender GA. *Great Moments in Pharmacy*. Detroit, Mich.: Northwood Institute Press; 1967.

In ancient Greece lived the Father of Botany, Theophrastus (about 300 B.C.). In addition to studying plants in general, Theophrastus made many observations about the medicinal qualities of herbs that have proven uncannily accurate.[3] Hippocrates of Cos formulated the theory of the four humors that parallel the four elements (air—blood, water—phlegm, earth—black bile, fire—yellow bile); he surmised that disease was caused by an imbalance of these bad humors. This led to centuries of medicine aimed at expelling from the ill person the offending, excess bad humors.[1]

Galenicals:
Historically used to refer to a class of pharmaceutical products that were compounded through mechanical means.

Galen (A.D. 130–200) practiced and taught medicine and pharmacy in ancient Rome. He developed principles of preparing and compounding medicinal agents that were followed for 1,500 years, and the word **galenicals**, derived from his name, is still used to refer to medicinal agents derived from natural sources that are prepared mechanically.[3] Galen and his followers sought to restore humoral balance within a patient by the use of medicines of opposing qualities (for example, inflammation would be treated with cucumber, a cool drug). He also drew from many available sources and attempted to organize and systematize the work begun by Hippocrates.[1]

Also from the Roman era came the patron saints of pharmacy and medicine, the twin brothers Damian and Cosmas. These devout Christians of Arab descent offered religious and medicinal solaces to those who came to them, until their twin careers were cut short in 303 by martyrdom. Damian, the apothecary, and Cosmas, the physician, became the patron saints of their closely allied professions.[3]

Pharmacy differentiates during the Middle Ages

Pharmaceutical knowledge—and the number of drugs available—grew considerably during the Middle Ages, thanks primarily to the Arabic world. Pharmacy as a separate activity began to develop, and privately owned pharmacies were established in Islamic lands. Medicine and pharmacy were for the first time separated.[1] The first known apothecary shop was opened in Baghdad in the eighth century, and the Muslims carried this concept into Europe during wars and other excursions into Africa, Spain, and southern France. The "Persian Galen," Ibn Sina (circa 980-1037), is known as Avicenna in the Western world. An intellectual giant, he was a physician, poet, philosopher, diplomat, and companion of Persian princes and rulers.[3] His Canon Medicinae brought together the best knowledge of the Greeks and Arabs into a single medical text.

Priests were also important in advancing the use of plants and other substances as medicines for patients during the Middle Ages.[1]

German Emperor Frederick II issued an edict in about 1240 that legally separated pharmacy from medicine in southern Italy and Sicily. Known as the Magna Carta of pharmacy, the edict contained three decrees:[1]

- The pharmaceutical profession was to be separated from the medical profession.
- The pharmaceutical profession should be supervised officially.
- Pharmacists should take an oath to prepare drugs reliably, according to skilled art, and in a uniform, suitable quality.

Each of these three requirements was critical in pharmacy's recognition by society and in later developments in the history of pharmacy.

Table 2.2 | World & Pharmacy Events During the Middle Ages

Year	Event	Year	Event
571–632	Mohammed.	1345	First apothecary shop in London.
711	Muslims invaded Spain.	1348–1350	Black Death.
768–814	Charlemagne.	1368	Ming Dynasty in China.
871–901	Alfred the Great.	1376	Board of Medical Examiners founded in London.
980–1036	Avicenna.	1440–1450	Invention of printing.
1066	Battle of Hastings.	1452–1519	Leonardo da Vinci.
1096–1272	Crusades.	1454	Gutenberg Bible printed.
1198	Hospital movement inaugurated by Innocent III.	1457	First medical publication (Gutenberg Purgation-Calendar).
1215	Magna Carta signed in Britain.	1478	Spanish Inquisition.
1227–1274	Thomas Aquinas.	1479	First edition of Avicenna printed.
1231	Medical school at Salerno.		
1271	Marco Polo began travels.		
1330	Gunpowder used in warfare.		
1336–1453	Hundred Years' War.		

Source: Adapted from Bender GA. *Great Moments in Pharmacy*. Detroit, Mich.: Northwood Institute Press; 1967.

Table 2.3 | World & Pharmacy Events During the Renaissance

Year	Event	Year	Event
1492	Columbus discovered America.	1660	Willis described puerperal fever.
1493–1541	Paracelsus.	1661	Malpighi published first account of capillary system (De pulmonibus).
1498	First official pharmacopeia (Florentine Receptario).	1661	Robert Boyle defined chemical elements and isolated acetone.
1509–1547	Reign of Henry VIII in England.	1661	Descartes published first treatise on physiology (De homine).
1517	Luther propounded his theses at Wittenberg.	1665	Newton discovered binomial theorem and law of gravitation.
1518	Royal College of Physicians founded in England.		
1524	Cortes erected hospital in Mexico.	1665	Great Plague of London.
1526	Paracelsus founded chemotherapy.	1666	Great Fire of London.
1540	English barbers and surgeons united as "Commonalty of the Barbers and Surgeons".	1669	Lower showed that venous blood takes up air in the lungs.
1543	Copernicus described revolution of Earth around sun.	1670	Malpighi discovered malpighian bodies in spleen and kidneys.
1543	English apothecaries legalized by act of Parliament.	1670	Willis discovered sweet taste of diabetic urine.
1558–1603	Reign of Elizabeth I.	1672	De Graaf described the graafian follicles in ovaries.
1561–1626	Francis Bacon.	1673	Leeuwenhoek began making microscopes.
1564–1616	Shakespeare.	1675	Leeuwenhoek discovered protozoa.
1564–1642	Galileo.	1682–1725	Peter the Great rules Russia.
1578–1657	William Harvey.	1683	Sydenham's treatise on gout published.
1584	Sir Walter Raleigh brought curare from Guiana.	1683	Leeuwenhoek described and sketched bacteria.
1590	Compound microscope invented.	1685–1750	Johann Sebastian Bach.
1604–1609	Galileo elucidated law of falling bodies.	1690	Locke's "Essay Concerning Human Understanding" published.
1606–1669	Rembrandt.		
1607	Settlement of Jamestown, Virginia.		
1609	Galileo turned telescope on the night sky.		
1609–1618	Kepler stated laws of planetary motion.		
1615–1616	Harvey lectured on circulation of blood.		
1617	Guild of Apothecaries of the City of London founded.		
1618	First edition of London Pharmacopoeia.		
1618–1648	Thirty Years' War.		
1620	Pilgrims landed at Plymouth, Massachusetts.		
1620	Van Helmont stressed chemical role of gastric juice in digestion.		
1622–1673	Molière.		
1628	Harvey published De Motu Cordis.		
1630–1638	Treatment of malarial fever with cinchona bark known in Peru.		
1632–1723	Antony van Leeuwenhoek (inventor of microscope).		
1636	Harvard College founded.		
1639	First hospital in Canada.		
1639–1650	Juan del Vigo introduced cinchona into Spain and Italy.		
1643	Sir Edward Greaves described typhus fever as a "new disease" in England.		
1648	Francesco Redi disproved theory of spontaneous generation.		
1654–1715	Reign of Louis XIV.		

Source: Adapted from Bender GA. *Great Moments in Pharmacy.* Detroit, Mich.: Northwood Institute Press; 1967.

The Renaissance: Pharmacists flourished too

Following the Middle Ages, many parts of European society re-examined the Greek and Roman tenets that they had held as fact. Thus, just as Copernicus challenged the Roman Catholic Church with his conclusion that the Earth revolved around the sun, pharmacists stood ready to consider new approaches to the prevention and treatment of disease.

Among the ideas that failed to stand up to closer scrutiny were the humoral pathology concepts of Hippocrates and their systemization by Galen and Avicenna.[1] The Swiss physician Parcelsus (1493–1541) was particularly important in that he introduced two ideas: Disease might be localized in a specific organ (rather than the entire body being affected), and such conditions could be treated internally using the chemical properties of medicinal agents, and some plants and other substances contained minute quantities of active chemicals, which could be removed by making tinctures, extracts, and essences.[1]

Professional associations of pharmacists emerged during the Renaissance, although some date back to the 1200s. In England, pharmacists had been under the jurisdiction of the Guild of Grocers, which monopolized the drug and spice trade. In 1617, King James I granted a charter recognizing the Society of Apothecaries of London.[3]

Other contemporaries in the sixteenth and seventeenth centuries believed that disease was produced through an imbalance of acid and alkaline substances in the body. The theory of iatrochemistry held that food was transformed by saliva and by a ferment secreted by the pancreas and that blood was made life giving through ferments from the gallbladder and lymph glands. These ideas provided convenient ways to categorize chemicals and drugs based on observed effects. Homeopathy, or treatment of disease with substances that produced similar symptoms as did the disease, also has its origins in the Renaissance period.[1]

Pharmacy in the United States: The early days

With the increased recognition and application of the scientific method in the 1700s and 1800s, modern pharmacy emerged. Progress in inorganic and organic chemistry, immunology, and chemotherapy began to change pharmacy from an empirically based profession to a knowledge-based one.[8]

Medicine and pharmacy in the New World were necessarily based on practices from Europe, but the Americas also adapted European practices to meet new needs and take advantage of new opportunities. Many new medicinal plants were exported from the New to the Old World, including guaicum, sassafras, copaiba, and balsam of Peru. Four distinct types of pharmacies could be found in the Americas by the eighteenth century: the dispensing physician, the apothecary shop, the general store, and the **wholesale druggist**. Dispensing physicians became less and less common, with the practice largely dying out around the end of the nineteenth century. Also of interest was that wholesale druggists of this period generally had a dispensing operation that operated like the apothecary shops.[1]

Wholesale druggists:
Intermediaries in the mercantile chain between manufacturers and retail outlets such as pharmacies.

Among the well-known pharmacists of the period were Christopher Marshall of Philadelphia; Hugh Mercer of Fredericksburg, Virginia; and Andrew Craigie, the apothecary general during the Revolutionary War.[1]

Table 2.4 | World & Pharmacy Events in the Eighteenth Century

Year	Event	Year	Event
1702	Stahl stated phlogiston theory.	1781–1826	René Théophile-Hyacinthe Laennec.
1718	Geoffroy published table of chemical relationships.	1783	Scheele discovered glycerin.
1719	Neumann reported thymol.	1783	First balloon ascension.
1721	Zabdiel Boylston inoculated for smallpox.	1783–1785	Lavoisier decomposed water and overthrew phlogiston theory.
1730	Frobenius described preparation of sulfuric ether.	1784	Scheele discovered citric acid.
1740	Thomas Dover developed "Dover's Powder".	1785	Minkelers first used illuminating gas in balloons.
1740–1786	Reign of Frederick the Great.	1785	Withering's treatise on the foxglove (digitalis) published.
1743	Red Cross arrangement at Battle of Dettingen.	1785	Scheele discovered malic acid.
1743–1794	Antoine Laurent Lavoisier.	1789	Klaproth discovered uranium and zirconium.
1749–1823	Edward Jenner.	1789–1799	French Revolution.
1750	Griffith Hughes gave classic account of yellow fever of 1715 (Barbados).	1792	Eli Whitney invented cotton gin.
1751	Pennsylvania Hospital established in Philadelphia with Jonathan Roberts as apothecary.	1793	Benjamin Bell differentiated between gonorrhea and syphilis.
1752	Medical Society founded in London.	1793	Lowitz discovered mono- and tri-chloroacetic acids.
1754–1757	Black discovered carbon dioxide.	1793–1794	Reign of Terror in France.
1755	John Morgan appointed as second apothecary at Pennsylvania Hospital.	1794	Lavoisier beheaded.
1767	Kay and Hargreaves invented spinning jenny (beginning of Industrial Revolution in England).	1794	Thomas Percival's code of medical ethics privately printed.
1768	Baumé created the hydrometer.	1795	Joseph B. Caventou, French pharmacist and scientist, born.
1768	Margraaf discovered hydrogen fluoride.	1795–1796	Société de Médecine de Paris founded.
1769–1821	Napoleon Bonaparte.	1796	Jenner vaccinated James Phipps.
1769	Scheele discovered tartaric acid.	1796	Lowitz prepared absolute alcohol and pure ether.
1770	First medical degree in United States conferred.	1796–1815	Napoleonic Wars.
1770–1827	Beethoven.	1797	Vauqueline discovered chromium.
1771–1774	Priestley and Scheele isolated oxygen ("dephlogisticated air").	1798	Jenner's Inquiry published.
1772	Priestley discovered nitrogen and nitrous oxide.	1799	Davy discovered anesthetic properties of laughing gas (nitrous oxide).
1773	Medical Society of London founded.	1800	Royal College of Surgeons of London chartered.
1773	Rouelle discovered urea.		
1774	Scheele discovered chlorine.		
1774	Wiegleb discovered myristic acid.		
1774	Rouelle defined chemical nature of a salt.		
1775	Lavoisier isolated and defined oxygen and defined an acid.		
1775	Andrew Craigie became first apothecary general of the United States.		
1775–1783	American Revolution.		
1777	Lavoisier described exchange of gases in respiration.		
1777	Scheele's experiments with silver chloride laid groundwork for photography.		
1778	William Brown published first American pharmacopeia, called the *Lititz Pharmacopeia*.		
1780	Benjamin Franklin invented bifocal lenses.		

Sources: Adapted from:

Sonnedecker G. *Kremers and Urdang's History of Pharmacy*. 4th ed. Philadelphia, Pa.: JB Lippincott Co; 1976.

LaWall CH. *Four Thousand Years of Pharmacy: An Outline History of Pharmacy and the Allied Sciences*. Philadelphia, Pa.: JB Lippincott Co; 1927.

Bender GA. *Great Moments in Pharmacy*. Detroit, Mich.: Northwood Institute Press; 1967.

Schmidt JE. *Medical Discoveries: Who and When*. Springfield, Ill.: Charles C Thomas; 1959.

Morton LT. *A Medical Bibliography (Garrison and Morton)*. London, England: Gower Publishing Co; 1983.

The New Encyclopaedia Britannica. 15th ed. Chicago: Encyclopaedia Britannica; 1991.

Pharmacy in the United States: The nineteenth century

Wholesale druggists and individual apothecaries began manufacturing and selling chemicals in the late 1700s; this was the basis for the later establishment of pharmaceutical companies. The world was changing from an agriculturally based economy to an industrial-based one, and pharmacy found itself caught in this shift. Some drugs could be manufactured using the newly discovered principles of chemistry. The smallpox vaccine of Jenner was proving that a person could be made immune to the ravages of infectious diseases. By the end of the nineteenth century, Koch's postulates had clearly proven the microbial basis of many diseases. A German chemist, Friedrich Wilhelm Adam Sertürner, first isolated the drug morphine from opium and thereby created recognition of the alkaloids as a distinct class of medicinal agents.[3]

In January 1820, an important meeting took place in the Senate chambers of the U.S. Capitol in Washington. There, delegates met to begin work on a national **pharmacopeia**. Thanks largely to the impetus provided by physician Lyman Spalding, the first *Pharmacopeia of the United States* was published that year, and it was the precursor to today's *United States Pharmacopeia*. The phrase "USP" at the end of drug names today denotes that the product complies with the standards set by the United States Pharmacopeial Convention, which continues to meet every 5 years to revise standards for the nation's drugs.[1]

> **Pharmacopeia:**
> Books listing drugs and other medical devices, including standards for their preparation and analysis, that are recognized by a governmental authority.

By the early 1800s, states were issuing licenses to apothecaries, often based on examination provided by the medical examining board; South Carolina was the first state to do so. In 1821, the Philadelphia College of Pharmacy (PCP) was founded, the first pharmacy organization in the United States. PCP soon provided classes for apprentices to learn pharmacy. The Philadelphia pharmacists were responding to two major threats: deterioration of the practice of pharmacy and discriminatory classification by the University of Pennsylvania medical faculty. Other schools followed quickly, often with help from PCP:[1]

- Massachusetts College of Pharmacy (1823)
- College of Pharmacy of the City (and County) of New York (1829)
- Maryland College of Pharmacy (1840)
- Cincinnati College of Pharmacy (1850)
- Chicago College of Pharmacy (1859)
- St. Louis College of Pharmacy (1864)

The school at Philadelphia became the heart of American pharmacy in the 1800s. In addition to setting the tone and direction for pharmacy education, its faculty and alumni were instrumental in the formation of APhA, founded as the American Pharmaceutical Association, during a convention of twenty delegates at PCP in 1852.

Indeed, in the rotunda of the APhA building in Washington today sits a statue of William Procter, Jr., of PCP, known as "The Father of American Pharmacy." Procter was an 1837 PCP graduate who served on the faculty for 20 years and for 30 years on the United States Pharmacopeial Convention's Committee on Revision. The first secretary of APhA, he was editor of the *American Journal of Pharmacy* for 22 years.

Table 2.5 | World & Pharmacy Events of the Nineteenth Century

Year	Event	Year	Event
1801–1820	Discovery and/or isolation of cerium, morphine, mannitol, cinchonic acid, iodine, lecithin, daphnin, narcotine, strychnine, brucine, colchicine, quinine, and cinchonine.	1841	Pharmaceutical Society of Great Britain founded.
		1842	Long introduced ether anesthesia.
		1843	O. W. Holmes pointed out contagiousness of puerperal fever.
1803–1808	Lewis and Clark expedition.	1845–1923	Wilhelm Conrad Röentgen.
1806	End of Holy Roman Empire.	1846	Morton introduced ether anesthesia.
1809	McDowell performed ovariotomy.	1846	J. Marion Sims devised vaginal speculum.
1810	Figuier published qualities of animal charcoal.	1847	American Medical Association organized.
1811	Valentine Seaman published first civilian American pharmacopeia at the New York Hospital.	1847	Helmholtz published treatise on conservation of energy.
		1847	Sir J. Y. Simpson introduced chloroform anesthesia.
1815–1878	Crawford W. Long.	1847	Semmelwise discovered pathogenesis of puerperal fever.
1816	Laennec invented stethoscope.	1848	Fehling introduced test for sugar in urine.
1818	Meissner coined the name alkaloid.	1848	Claude Bernard demonstrated that glycogen is synthesized in the liver.
1819	Braconnet obtained grape sugar, treating sawdust with sulfuric acid.	1849	J. Marion Sims successfully operated for vesico-vaginal fistula.
1819–1868	William Thomas Green Morton.	1850	Claude Bernard published studies on arrow poisons.
1820	First U. S. Pharmacopeia published.	1850	Fehling developed solution for detection of sugar.
1820–1910	Florence Nightingale.	1851	Helmholtz invented ophthalmoscope.
1821–1840	Discovery and/or isolation of caffeine, iodoform, pectin, pectic acid, bromine, ethyl bromide, aluminum, santonin, chloroform, coniine, codeine, narceine, thebaine, dextrin, carbolic acid, aniline, and pure chloroform.	1851–1902	Walter Reed.
		1851–1853	Pravaz introduced hypodermic needle.
		1852	American Pharmaceutical Association founded (now American Pharmacists Association).
1821	Döbereiner discovered the process of catalysis.	1853–1856	Crimean War, during which Florence Nightingale founded the modern nursing profession.
1821	Philadelphia College of Pharmacy founded.	1854–1915	Paul Ehrlich.
1822–1895	Louis Pasteur.	1859	Darwin's Origin of Species published.
1825	Publication of the *American Journal of Pharmacy*, first professional pharmacy periodical in English.	1860	Pasteur demonstrated presence of bacteria in air.
		1861–1865	American Civil War.
1827–1912	Lord Joseph Lister.	1865	Lister introduced antiseptic treatment of wounds.
1829	Dagueree introduced photography.	1865	Gregor Mendel published memoirs about plant hybridity.
1829	Tuéry demonstrated antidotal properties of charcoal.	1865	First International Pharmaceutical Congress convened in Brunswick, Germany.
1830–1848	Reign of Louis Philippe.	1866	A. J. Ångström introduced ångström units.
1832	British Medical Association founded.	1867	Lister introduced antiseptic surgery.
1832–1905	Albert B. Prescott.	1868	Clinical thermometer introduced.
1833	Johannes Müller's treatise on physiology published.	1869	Virchow urged medical inspection of schools.
1833	William Beaumont published experiments on gastric digestion.	1870	Fritsch and Hitzig investigated the localization of function of brain.
1835	Berzelius coined the term catalysis.	1870–1871	Franco–Prussian War (test of vaccination).
1837	Gerhard differentiated between typhus and typhoid fevers.	1871	Lister noted antibiotic phenomena.
1837	Victoria became Queen of England.	1876	Koch obtained pure cultures of anthrax bacilli on artificial media.
1839	Schwann published treatise on cell theory.	1876	Bell patented telephone.
1840	Henle published statement of germ theory of communicable diseases.	1878	Von Basch measured blood pressure with sphygmomanometer.
1841–1860	Discovery and/or isolation of niobium, cocaine from coca leaves, aniline dyes, and pure cocaine.		

Table 2.5 | World & Pharmacy Events of the Nineteenth Century, *continued*

Year	Event	Year	Event
1878	Edison invented platinum-wire (incandescent) electric lightbulb.	1897	Emil Fischer synthesized caffeine, theobromine, xanthine, guanine, and adenine.
1879	Billings and Fletcher started Index Medicus.	1897	Ehrlich stated the side chain theory of immunity.
1881	Pasteur produced anthrax vaccine.	1898	P. and M. Curie discovered radium.
1883	Susan Hayhurst became first woman to graduate from the Philadelphia College of Pharmacy; she was in charge of the pharmacy of the Woman's Hospital of Philadelphia for 3 decades.	1898	Dreser introduced heroin.
		1898	National Association of Retail Druggists (now National Community Pharmacists Association) founded.
1885	Pasteur introduced rabies vaccine.	1899	Walter Reed and others demonstrated mosquito transmission of yellow fever.
1886	Limousin developed glass ampuls for storage of hypodermic solutions.	1899	Dreser introduced aspirin.
1889	Behring introduced antitoxins.	1900	Conference of Pharmaceutical Faculties founded (now American Association of Colleges of Pharmacy).
1895	Röentgen discovered X-rays.		
1895	Marconi introduced wireless telegraph.		

Source: Adapted from Bender GA. *Great Moments in Pharmacy*. Detroit, Mich.: Northwood Institute Press; 1967.

During the latter half of the nineteenth century, pharmacy schools operated primarily as finishing schools; pharmacy apprentices with several years' experience in apothecary shops would attend school for a limited amount of time before becoming licensed pharmacists. A physician-chemist at the University of Michigan changed that. Albert B. Prescott believed that the scientific foundation of pharmacy should be laid first through didactic educational programs and only then should the student attempt to learn the practical side of the trade through an apprenticeship. Prescott, dean of pharmacy at the University of Michigan, went up against organized pharmacy with his beliefs, and for it he was rejected as a delegate at the 1871 APhA convention in St. Louis. But time proved him right, and by the turn of the century, most schools began adopting his model. He served as president of APhA in 1899–1900 and of the predecessor organization of the American Association of Colleges of Pharmacy in 1900.[9]

Twentieth-century pharmacy: A business or a profession?

William Procter, the influential PCP faculty member, was prescient when he identified what would become a chief problem for twentieth-century pharmacists. As quoted by Hepler,[8] Procter wrote in 1858:

[I]f the preparation of medicines is taken from the apothecary and he becomes merely the dispenser of them, his business is shorn of half its dignity and importance, and he relapses into a simple shopkeeper.

By the beginning of the twentieth century, the pharmaceutical industry had begun to make an impact on the daily lives of pharmacists. More and more products were produced ready to dispense, and problems with adulteration and quackery caused the U.S. Congress to pass the Pure Food and Drug Act in 1906 (see Chapter 7). In Germany, new discoveries in organic chemistry were making possible the increased rational design of drugs (as well as creating horrors during World War I because of the use of lethal nerve gases).

Table 2.6 | World & Pharmacy Events, 1901–1950

Year	Event	Year	Event
1901	Landsteiner discovered blood groups (isoagglutination).	1938	Hahn developed device for nuclear fission.
1901	Awarding of Nobel prizes began.	1939–1945	World War II.
1902–1903	Jensen propagated cancer through several generations of mice.	1939	Florey and Chain developed penicillin to stage of therapeutic use.
1903	Wright brothers made successful flight with airplane.	1939	More than 150 different kinds of synthetic materials were known.
1904–1914	Panama Canal built.	1940	Karl Link discovered dicumarol.
1906	Pure Food and Drugs Act passed in the United States.	1940	Landsteiner and Wiener discovered Rhesus factor in blood.
1910	Abraham Flexner published survey of medical schools and education.	1940	American College of Apothecaries founded.
Early 1900s	Several hormones and vitamins identified.	1942	Atomic energy released and controlled in first nuclear chain reaction.
1914–1918	World War I.	1942	First jet aircraft tested.
1914	Flexner stated that pharmacy was not a profession.	1942	American Society of Hospital (now Health-System) Pharmacists founded.
1915	Twort reported on bacteriophages.	1943	Penicillin production began.
1916	Bull introduced antitoxin for gas gangrene.	1944	Waksman announced discovery of streptomycin.
1918	Surgeon General ruled that pharmacy was not a profession.	1944	Synthesis of quinine.
1918–1919	Spanish influenza pandemic.	1945	Worldwide antimalarial campaign using DDT.
1921	Banting and Best isolated insulin.	1945	United Nations formed.
1925	First state association of hospital pharmacists formed, in California.	1946	Penicillin produced synthetically.
1926	E. L. Kennaway extracted the first known cancer-causing chemical, 3,4-benzpyrene.	1947	Chloramphenicol discovered.
1926	Förster developed the brain-function chart.	1948	Farber found that antagonists to folic acid alleviated leukemia.
1927	Lindbergh crossed the Atlantic in airplane alone.	1948	World Health Organization founded.
1928	Alexander Fleming discovered penicillin.	1948	Kinsey report on sexual behavior of the human male.
1928	Forssmann performed the first heart catheterization.	1948	200-inch telescope installed at Mount Palomar Observatory.
1929	Worldwide stock market crash; beginning of Great Depression.	1950–1953	Korean conflict.
1931	Development of electron microscope.		
1932	Chadwick, Joliot-Curie, and Urey discovered, respectively, the neutron, positron, and heavy hydrogen.		
1932	Zernike developed the phase-contrast microscope.		
1933	Hitler rose to power in Germany.		
1935	Trefouel, Nitti, and Bovet discovered Prontosil's action to be caused by sulfanilamide.		
1935	Kendall and Reichstein isolated cortisone.		
1935	Stanley discovered the virus agent of tobacco mosaic, a "living" molecule.		
1935	Nucleic acids found to be the principal components of viruses and genes.		
1936	Hospital pharmacy section of American Pharmaceutical (now Pharmacists) Association formed.		
1937	Sulfonamide therapy for gonorrhea introduced.		
1938	Federal Food, Drug and Cosmetic Act passed, increasing federal oversight of drugs.		
1938	Hess discovered regulatory function of the midbrain.		

Source: Adapted from Bender GA. *Great Moments in Pharmacy*. Detroit, Mich.: Northwood Institute Press; 1967.

As the century progressed, the pharmaceutical industry became stronger. The dramatic acceleration came during and following World War II. The military had an urgent need for penicillin, which had lain dormant in Fleming's laboratory for 10 years. The technology, scientific knowledge, and need were present all at once, and the post–World War II pharmaceutical industry began producing drugs that were much more powerful and specific than those available previously.

The effect of this on pharmacists was twofold: The art of **compounding** rapidly became less important, as most prescriptions could be filled with manufactured dosage forms, and the knowledge about the drugs, their mechanisms of action, and their side effects became much more complicated.

Pharmacy had already encountered problems during the first half of the twentieth century in maintaining or gaining recognition as a profession. In 1918, the Surgeon General refused to recognize pharmacy as such, which meant that pharmacists could not be commissionable officers in the Armed Forces, as were professionals such as physicians and engineers. Pharmacy had responded in 1932 by standardizing pharmacy school curricula as 4-year programs leading to attainment of the bachelor of science degree in pharmacy.[8] This was not enough, however, and pharmacists remained enlisted personnel during World War II.

Consequently, the end of World War II found a pharmacy profession in an emaciated state. As Brushwood wrote during the celebration of APhA's sesquicentennial, "By 1952 pharmacists had become what they sought to be: respected custodians of the nation's drug supply, at the tail end of the chain of distribution. This is an important role, but not a fulfillment of the promise of the profession in 1902, when an expansive patient-oriented practice appeared to be developing."[10] Because pharmacists were not recognized as professionals by the military,[11] schools had been decimated by conscription during the war. Pharmacists of that period found that much of their knowledge and many of their skills were rendered useless by the new technologies of pharmaceutical industry. A major challenge for the leaders of pharmacy lay in store during the latter half of the twentieth century.

Compounding:
The preparation of prescriptions specifically for a patient based on an individualized drug order from a prescriber.

REFERENCES

1. Sonnedecker G. *Kremers and Urdang's History of Pharmacy*. 4th ed. Philadelphia, Pa.: JB Lippincott Co; 1976. (Copies of this book are available from the American Institute of the History of Pharmacy, http://pharmacy.wisc.edu/aihp/order-publications.)
2. LaWall CH. *Four Thousand Years of Pharmacy: An Outline History of Pharmacy and the Allied Sciences*. Philadelphia, Pa.: JB Lippincott Co; 1927.
3. Bender GA. *Great Moments in Pharmacy*. Detroit, Mich.: Northwood Institute Press; 1967. (Note: This book contains reprints of the Parke–Davis History of Pharmacy oil paintings; however, it is not the best source of specific historical information.)
4. American Pharmacists Association. Great moments in pharmacy (painting series). www.pharmacist. com/great-moments-pharmacy-painting-series. Accessed June 16, 2016.
5. Griffenhagen GB. Great moments in pharmacy: development of the Robert Thom series depicting pharmacy's history. *J Am Pharm Assoc*. 2002;42(2):170–82.
6. Griffenhagen GB. *Pharmaceutical Philately*. Johnstown, Pa.: American Topical Association; 1990.
7. Cowen DL, Helfand WH. *Pharmacy: An Illustrated History*. New York: Abrams; 1990.

8. Hepler CD. The third wave in pharmaceutical education: the clinical movement. *Am J Pharm Educ.* 1987;51(4):369–85.

9. Manasse HR Jr. Innovation, confrontation, and perseverance: Albert B. Prescott's legacy to pharmaceutical education in America. *Pharm Hist.* 1973;15(1):22–8.

10. Brushwood DB. Governance of pharmacy, 1902-52. *J Am Pharm Assoc.* 2001;41(3):376–7.

11. Worthen DB. Carl Thomas Durham (1892-1974): pharmacy's representative. *J Am Pharm Assoc.* 2005;45(2):295–8.

Chapter 3

Pharmacy Reborn: From Clinical Services to Pharmacists' Patient Care Services

Abir A. (Abby) Kahaleh

As reflected in the history presented in Chapter 2, societies have for centuries devised systems to provide solutions to people's problems. In the caves of thousands of years ago, our predecessors probably had job descriptions very similar to one another: find food, prepare it, protect themselves and their family from harm, and reproduce. Life was difficult, but the jobs were all about the same.

As the human species evolved, specialized tasks became more the norm. Some people were farmers, whereas others worked with newly discovered metals. Curing the infirmities of the ill became the main activity of some people, and discovering grand schemes of making war motivated others.

For centuries, people continued to develop more and more specialized roles, and a person in need would seek the materials, services, advice, or expertise of his or her neighbors in a relatively restricted community. Little need existed for any formal recognition of specialized expertise because most people knew each other and knew for what each could be relied upon. Travel was difficult, leaving most people circumscribed to a small geographic area throughout their disease- and war-shortened lives.

However, as the Middle Ages began to wane, people became more mobile, and cities began to grow. People no longer knew all their neighbors. Jobs became more specialized. In response, a variety of alliances and organizations of merchants and businesspeople involved in similar activities began to develop. These organizations were often formed with self-serving interests in mind, such as to limit competition by requiring all parties to abide by certain standards. But they also served a useful purpose in that standards began to develop by which various trades began to practice. Some of these sponsoring organizations evolved into professional associations, others into labor unions, and some into trade groups.

By the eighteenth century, many of these standards or restrictions had been adopted by governmental bodies, giving the force of law to the previously voluntary requirements. The Industrial Revolution, generally considered to occur from the late 1700s until the mid-twentieth century, accelerated this change, as did the rapid pace of scientific discoveries. Jobs became highly specialized, and the tasks performed by a given group of workers could not be easily completed by those outside the field.

Occupations vs. professions

As society recognized the increasing complexity of some jobs, people began to differentiate further between a work activity that was a job, a lifelong or long-term devotion to an occupation, and the specialized knowledge and unique requirements of a profession.

Learning Objectives

Upon completion of this chapter, the reader should be able to:

1. Identify historic publications that shaped the profession by expanding the clinical role of pharmacists.

2. Describe pharmaceutical care, medication therapy management, and pharmacists' patient care services.

3. Highlight critical factors that led to the current role of pharmacists in public health.

"Pharmaceutical care gives us hope that our profession can restore its past greatness, not by our becoming chemists again, but rather by our making a commitment to outcomes that are valuable beyond price to our patients, in a health care environment that is being stood on its head by rapid change."

— Charles D. Hepler, in "Four Virtues for the Future," 1997 Remington Lecture

Differentiating between an occupation and a profession has occupied many sociologists' minds for decades. Charles D. Hepler, a pharmacist and pharmacy professor at the University of Florida, wrote extensively about pharmacy and its professional status in the 1980s and 1990s. Let's look at some of his conclusions.

Hepler[1] relies on the basic observations of Magali Sarfatti Larsen[2] in characterizing a profession. Three basic characteristics have become the hallmarks of professions:[1]
- The services offered are closely linked to major human values, such as health, property, or religion.
- The services require a degree of knowledge, skill, and understanding beyond those possessed by ordinary people of the day and beyond a layman's ability to evaluate (for example, the accuracy of a diagnosis or the purity of a prescription).
- The services are inherently personal or individualized in nature, meaning that they cannot be readily standardized or mass produced.

These three requirements surely prove that pharmacy of the nineteenth century was a profession, Hepler concluded. Pharmacy has always concerned itself with health. One has to have special training—indeed, special tools—to determine what ingredients are present in a tablet or tincture. And a brief review of the prescription files crumbling from age in an old pharmacy will show that few patients received the same medications; medicaments were highly individualized, and the pharmacist compounded many prescriptions specifically for a patient immediately before dispensing.[1,3]

However, what about pharmacy of the twentieth century? Amendments to the Federal Food, Drug, and Cosmetic Act of 1938 required pharmaceutical manufacturers to spend millions of dollars in premarket testing of drugs, and advances in technology allowed mass production of ready-to-dispense tablets, capsules, suppositories, liquids, and injectables. Prescriptions became so standardized that some pharmaceutical companies gave physicians preprinted prescription pads complete with drug name, quantity to dispense, and directions. As Hepler noted, the only individualization was the patient's name and the prescription number, and "the complexity of most pharmaceutical service was reduced in the public mind, and often in reality, to the infamous sequence of counting, pouring, licking, and sticking."[3]

Pharmacy, always plagued by the image of the merchant interested primarily in moving the drug products, thus had come perilously close to losing any valid status as a profession.

Pharmaceutical care as reprofessionalization

Luckily, the same development that threatened pharmacy—the industrialization of the pharmaceutical industry in the first half of the twentieth century—also provided the profession with a valuable opportunity.

Efficacy:
The ability of a drug to produce desired therapeutic effects.

Any cursory review of pharmacology or medical books from just a few decades ago quickly demonstrates that **efficacious** drugs were few and far between. Although the explosion in knowledge of chemicals described in Chapter 2 had provided some powerful agents, many of the drugs were merely palliative. Antibiotics were not yet available, the pathophysiology of many disease states was not well understood, and the best many patients could hope for was relief from suffering until the disease took its course.

In the 1950s, scientists began to make major strides in understanding biological systems; remember that it was not until 1953 that DNA was proven to be the genetic material of living organisms. Just as physics had been advanced in the 1600s, and chemistry made great strides in the 1800s and early 1900s, the time for biology came in the 1900s. Finally, medical scientists understood specifically what underlying metabolic or genetic defect caused certain diseases, and with this knowledge powerful new drugs were identified or in some cases created to cure the conditions (see Table 3.1).

Table 3.1 | Pharmacy & World Events, 1951–Present

Year	Event	Year	Event
1951	Durham-Humphrey Amendments to Food, Drug, and Cosmetic Act passed by U.S. Congress, more clearly identifying drugs that required prescribing by a licensed medical practitioner.	1974	Restriction endonucleases discovered, thus permitting genetic engineering and sparking the biotechnology revolution.
1951	Ludwig Gross showed virus transmission of leukemia in mice.	1975	Supreme Court decision in Portland Retail Druggists Association v. Abbott Laboratories et al. limits distribution of specially priced pharmaceutical drugs by nonprofit entities.
1951	J. André-Thomas developed the heart-lung machine.		
1951	International Pharmacopoeia published by World Health Organization.	1975	ASHP formed special-interest groups to meet the diverse needs of emerging practice areas.
1951	Effect of fluoride on dental caries discovered.	1975	Millis Commission issues report on the future of pharmacy.
1952	Reserpine discovered.	1976	The Board of Pharmaceutical (now Pharmacy) Specialties is formed as an autonomous division within APhA. It has since approved as specialties Nuclear Pharmacy (1978), Nutrition Support Pharmacy (1988), Pharmacotherapy (1988), Psychiatric Pharmacy (1994), Oncology Pharmacy (1996), Ambulatory Care Pharmacy (2009), Pediatric Pharmacy (2013), and Critical Care Pharmacy (2013).
1952	First open-heart operation by Baily.		
1952	First hydrogen bomb explosion.		
1955	Jonas Salk developed polio vaccine.		
1957	First space satellite launched.		
1959	Polonski described the function of DNA.		
1960	Introduction of the laser.		
1961	First manned space travel.	1979	American College of Clinical Pharmacy founded.
1962	Drug amendments passed, requiring efficacy of new drugs (in addition to a previous requirement of safety).	1980	Food and Drug Administration (FDA) required mandatory patient package inserts for 10 major drugs and drug classes during the waning days of the Carter administration (the regulations were rescinded in 1981 by the Reagan administration).
1963	American Society of Health-System Pharmacists (ASHP) begins accreditation of hospital pharmacy residencies.		
1963	Lasers used in medicine.		
1963	Oxytocic drugs used in obstetrics.	1981	American Association of Colleges of Pharmacy (AACP) rejected PharmD as entry-level degree.
1963	John F. Kennedy assassinated.		
1964	Pharmacist Hubert H. Humphrey elected vice president of the United States.	1981	Michigan Pharmacists Association began certifying pharmacy technicians based on examination.
1964–73	Americans involved in combat in Vietnam.	1983	APhA president William S. Apple died.
1966	Ninth Floor Project begins at University of California–San Francisco, leading to clinical pharmacy movement.	1984	First Pharmacy in the 21st Century conference held.
1967	First human heart transplanted by Christiaan Barnard.	1985	Directions in Clinical Pharmacy Practice conference held at Hilton Head, South Carolina.
1969	American Society of Consultant Pharmacists founded.	1989	Accreditation Council for Pharmacy Education proposed elimination of the BS Pharmacy degree, leading to establishment of PharmD as entry-level degree for pharmacy.
1969	Americans land on moon.		
1970	Bureau of Narcotics and Dangerous Drugs reorganized as Drug Enforcement Administration.		
1972	U.S. postage stamp issued in honor of pharmacy.	1989	Academy of Managed Care Pharmacy founded.
1974	Richard Nixon resigned presidency as a result of Watergate scandal.		

continued on page 24

Table 3.1 | Pharmacy & World Events, 1951–Present, *continued*

Year	Event	Year	Event
1989–90	Congress first passed but then repealed legislation covering outpatient prescription drugs for the elderly.	2001	September 11 terrorist attacks.
1990	Congress passed amendments to the Omnibus Budget Reconciliation Act requiring pharmacists to offer medication counseling to Medicaid prescriptions when they are dispensed the first time. Many state boards of pharmacy extended the requirement to include all patients.	2001	Pharmacists fall to fourth in trust/ethics poll, tied with police and trailing firefighters, the U.S. military, and nurses.
		2003	Iraqi War begins.
		2003	APhA changes its name to American Pharmacists Association.
1992	APhA, ASHP, and AACP conducted the Scope of Pharmacy Practice project, with a goal of redefining the typical activities of pharmacists and technicians.	2003	Medicare Part D created by Congress covering outpatient prescription drugs.
		2006	Number of certified pharmacy technicians (CPhTs) passes 250,000 mark, exceeding number of licensed pharmacists.
1994	ASHP changes its name to the American Society of Health-System Pharmacists.	2008	Permanent CPhT billing codes for medication therapy management services take effect.
1995	Formation of the Pharmacy Technician Certification Board; first administration of a national pharmacy technician certification examination.	2010	Affordable Care Act signed into law following year-long national debate over health care reform.
1997	Joseph A. Oddis retires after 37 years as chief executive officer at ASHP.	2012	Products for injection prepared at a Boston-area compounding pharmacy caused illness in more than 800 patients and deaths in 64 patients, leading to federal legislation and increased regulation of this part of pharmacy practice.
1997	Pharmacists in Asheville, North Carolina, begin providing pharmaceutical care to patients with diabetes in what would become known as the Asheville Project.	2013	Pharmacy organizations launch effort to achieve recognition of pharmacists as providers eligible for payment under federal Medicare statutes.
1998	Pharmacists named most trusted professionals in United States for 10th year in a row.	2015	Pharmacy Technician Certification Board celebrates 20th anniversary; number of CPhTs at 550,000, compared with 290,000 pharmacists in early 2016.
1999	Internet pharmacies become common on the World Wide Web.		
1999	FDA begins requiring patient package inserts with some prescription drugs.	2016	New ACPE standard for education of pharmacists becomes effective. The number of colleges and schools of pharmacy reached 135, and the number of student pharmacists was approaching 65,000.
2000	ACPE regulations for the new PharmD degree became effective.		
2001	Robert R. Courtney, a Kansas City pharmacist, is arrested for providing to physicians for cancer patients intravenous solutions that contained little or no medication.		

Source: Adapted in part from Bender GA. *Great Moments in Pharmacy*. Detroit, Mich.: Northwood Institute Press; 1967.

In addition, thousands of compounds were tested for antibacterial, antifungal, and antiviral activity in the ensuing decades. Despite the current concern over antibiotic resistance, myriad commercially available antibiotics are available for treating diseases that regularly killed and debilitated people only half a century ago. Some people attribute the so-called sexual revolution of the 1960s not only to the availability of oral contraceptives ("birth control pills") but just as much to the marketing of antibiotics that could cure sexually transmitted bacterial infections. In short, new drugs were changing the world.

In the late 1950s and 1960s, astute pharmacists such as Donald C. Brodie of the University of California–San Francisco, Donald E. Francke of the University of Michigan, and Paul F. Parker of the University of Kentucky began to conceptualize a new role for pharmacists that would involve the specialized provision of information about these powerful new agents that were beginning to reach the market. As it came to be known, the clinical pharmacy movement sought to create a role for pharmacists in the provision of patient-specific drug information or advice to physicians and other members of the health care team.

Hepler has identified three simultaneous trends that served as the basis for the clinical pharmacy movement: **drug information**; **drug distribution**, especially **decentralized** programs in hospitals; and teaching and research programs in **pharmacology** and **biopharmaceutics**.[3] These three currents combined for the first time in the famous 1966 Ninth Floor Project at the University of California–San Francisco, in which faculty sought to find a way to train students for a role that did not previously exist. The problem was stated this way:[4]

[Although] the concept of the pharmacist as a drug consultant was stressed and attempts were made to instruct the student in how his pharmaceutical knowledge related to patient care … the faculty had no opportunity to test their techniques of instruction for there was no laboratory at that time where the students could put their training into practice.

The project began in September 1966 with the following goals:[4]
- To develop a hospital floor–based pharmaceutical service that would provide maximal patient **safety** in the utilization of drugs.
- To charge the pharmacist with the responsibility for all phases of drug distribution, except the administration of medication to the patient.
- To provide an unbiased and easily available source of reliable drug information (the pharmacist) and to disseminate information according to the needs of professional personnel.
- To provide clinical experience for interns and residents and other qualified pharmacy students in hospital pharmacy.
- To design and conduct studies in cooperation with the physician and nurse so that a full evaluation may be obtained of institutional pharmacy service within the framework of the team approach to patient care.

All of these roles were radical departures from prior functions of pharmacists. But gradually, the worth of such services took hold, and schools of pharmacy across the country began to create a demand for clinical pharmacy services by placing pharmacy faculty in acute-care institutions and giving medical residents and interns a taste of what highly motivated and competent pharmacists could accomplish.

The publication of *Drug Intelligence and Clinical Pharmacy* (now *Annals of Pharmacotherapy*) began in 1967, and two pharmacy therapeutics textbooks came out of San Francisco in 1972. By 1974, the federal government recognized a clinical role for pharmacists when it began requiring the pharmacist to conduct monthly **drug-regimen reviews** of residents in skilled-care **nursing homes**, thanks to the efforts of pharmacists such as George F. Archambault, Richard S. Berman, and other leaders of the fledgling American Society of Consultant Pharmacists.

Thus, the clinical pharmacy movement created the opportunity for pharmacy to continue as a profession worthy of the respect and trust of its patients: clinical pharmacy was involved in the health care of patients, it required specialized knowledge and skills, and it was individualized.

Drug information:
A service provided by pharmacists to other health professionals or to the public in which basic or detailed information about drugs is provided.

Decentralized drug distribution:
Systems in hospitals of distributing drugs to patients in which pharmacy services are located in several locations near patient care areas rather than in one central pharmacy.

Pharmacology:
The study of the action of drugs in biological systems.

Biopharmaceutics:
The study of a drug's physical and chemical properties as they relate to the effects of the drug on the body (absorption, distribution, and metabolism or elimination).

Safety:
The ability of a drug not to produce harmful or deleterious side effects or adverse reactions.

Drug-regimen review:
A clinical pharmacy service provided to residents of nursing homes in which pharmacists review the drug therapy of residents and provide suggestions to physicians about drug selection, duplication, necessity, adverse effects, or monitoring.

Nursing homes:
Facilities that provide residential care and health care to residents who live in them. Residents are typically deficient in one or more activities of daily living: ambulating, feeding, bathing, or toileting.

Affirmation of the trend: The Millis Report

In 1975, the American Association of Colleges of Pharmacy commissioned a study of pharmacy by a 12-member group headed by Dr. John Millis, a nonpharmacist educator who had recently completed a study of physician education. Known commonly as the Millis Commission, the group issued its findings in a 161-page report called *Pharmacists for the Future: The Report of the Study Commission on Pharmacy.*

The commission made 14 recommendations, which are paraphrased or summarized in Table 3.2. Among the changes in pharmacy and pharmacy education as a direct result of the Millis Commission were the following:

- Acceleration of development of clinical sites for pharmacy school faculty
- Development of a national examination for licensure of pharmacists, now called the NAPLEX® (North American Pharmacist Licensure Examination®)
- Increased movement toward making pharmacy a knowledge-based clinical profession
- Creation of a small number of clinical scientists programs in schools of pharmacy at the doctor of philosophy level
- Creation of a Board of Pharmaceutical Specialties within APhA to recognize specialty practices in pharmacy and certify individuals in those specialties

However, as Hepler has noted,[3] the Millis Report failed to produce a real spark in shifting pharmacy dramatically and irreversibly toward its desired goals. Unlike some previous similar reports in pharmacy or medicine, the Millis Report did not outline specific changes in pharmacy school curricula or give a blueprint for the future. It provided only external recognition for the advances made by pharmacy as a clinical profession.

Hepler and Strand raise the stakes with pharmaceutical care

The clinical pharmacy movement continued in the 1980s. Two new journals were published: *Pharmacotherapy* was founded in 1981 by the late Russell R. Miller, a clinical scientist of the ilk envisioned by the Millis Commission, and *Clinical Pharmacy* was published by the American Society of Hospital Pharmacists from 1982 through 1993. A third textbook in the clinical pharmacy field, *Pharmacotherapy: A Pathophysiologic Approach*, was first published in 1989.

The term *pharmacotherapist* was chosen to designate specialists in clinical pharmacy when the Board of Pharmaceutical Specialties recognized this part of practice in 1988. Certified pharmacotherapy specialists carry the initials *BCPS* following their names.

But Hepler began to conclude that the clinical pharmacy and pharmacotherapy movement was not the sole answer to pharmacy's problems. Beginning at the 1985 Directions for Clinical Practice in Pharmacy (called commonly the Hilton Head conference because of its South Carolina meeting site), Hepler expounded on the notion that pharmacists had to do more than just try to control the use of drugs. Hepler preached that they had to take responsibility for the care provided to patients through the clinical use of drugs. In 1987, he first applied the term *pharmaceutical care*[3] in describing what he and colleague Linda Strand called these new self-actualizing roles for pharmacists.[5]

Table 3.2 | **Summary of the Concepts, Findings, and Recommendations of the Study Commission on Pharmacy**

1. Among deficiencies in the health care system is the unavailability of adequate information for those who consume, prescribe, dispense, and administer drugs. Pharmacists are health professionals who could make an important contribution to the health care system of the future by providing information about drugs to consumers and health professionals. Education and training of pharmacists must be developed to meet these important responsibilities.

2. Pharmacy should be conceived basically as a knowledge system that renders a health service by concerning itself with understanding drugs and their effects upon people and animals.

3. A pharmacist must be defined as an individual who is engaged in one of the steps of a system called pharmacy. … A pharmacist is characterized by the common denominator of drug knowledge and the differentiated additional knowledge and skill required by his or her particular role.

4. The system of pharmacy must be described as being both effective and efficient in developing, manufacturing, and distributing drug products. However, it cannot be described at present as either effective or efficient in developing, organizing, and distributing knowledge and information about drugs.

5. Major attention should be given to the problems of drug information—specifically in defining who needs to know, what that person needs to know, and how these needs can best be met with speed and economy.

6. Despite the real and multifaceted differentiation in the practice roles of pharmacists, all pharmacists must possess a common body of knowledge, skill, attitudes, and behavior. The objectives of pharmacy education must be stated in terms of both the common knowledge and skill and the differentiated and/or additional knowledge and skill required for specific practice roles.

7. The Study Commission recommends the following three component educational objectives for pharmacy education:
   a. The mastery of the knowledge and the acquisition of the skills common to all of the roles of pharmacy practice.
   b. The mastery of the additional knowledge and the acquisition of the additional skills needed for those differentiated roles that require additional pharmacy knowledge and experience.
   c. The mastery of the additional knowledge and the acquisition of the additional skills needed for those differentiated roles that require additional knowledge and skill other than pharmacy.

8. Every school of pharmacy should promptly find the ways and means to provide appropriate practice opportunities for its faculty members having clinical teaching responsibilities so that they may serve as effective role models for their students.

9. The curricula of the schools of pharmacy should be based on the competencies desired for their graduates rather than upon the basis of knowledge available in the several relevant sciences.

10. The greatest weakness of the schools of pharmacy is a lack of an adequate number of clinical scientists who can relate their specialized scientific knowledge to the development of practice skills.

11. Pharmacy is a knowledge system in which chemical substances and people called patients interact. Needed and optimally effective drug therapy results only when drugs and those who consume them are fully understood. One of the first steps in reviewing the educational program of a college of pharmacy should be weighing the relative emphasis given to the physical and biological sciences in the curriculum for the first professional pharmacy degree.

12. Those schools of pharmacy with adequate resources should develop, in addition to the first professional degree, programs of instruction at the graduate and advanced professional level for more differentiated roles of pharmacy practice.

13. The optimal environment for pharmacy education is the university health science center, for the full range of knowledge, skill, and practice can be found there. However, the commission does not believe that it is practical or in the public interest to recommend that all colleges of pharmacy must be so located. Alternative arrangements, if effectively used, can provide an acceptable environment for the education of students at the baccalaureate level.

14. All aspects of the credentialing of pharmacists and pharmacy education would be enhanced by the services of a National Board of Pharmacy Examiners, created by joint action of the National Association of Boards of Pharmacy, the American Council on Pharmaceutical Education, and the American Association of Colleges of Pharmacy.

Source: Study Commission on Pharmacy. Pharmacists for the Future. Ann Arbor, Mich.: Health Administration Press; 1975:139–43.

Table 3.3 | Definition of Pharmaceutical Care

Pharmaceutical care is the responsible provision of drug therapy for the purpose of achieving definite outcomes that improve a patient's quality of life. These outcomes are (a) cure of a disease; (b) elimination or reduction of a patient's symptomatology; (c) arresting or slowing of a disease process; and (d) preventing a disease or symptomatology.

Pharmaceutical care involves the process through which a pharmacist cooperates with a patient and other professionals in designing, implementing, and monitoring a therapeutic plan that will produce specific therapeutic outcomes for the patient. This in turn involves three major functions: identifying potential and actual drug-related problems; resolving actual drug-related problems; and preventing potential drug-related problems.

Pharmaceutical care is a necessary element of health care and should be integrated with other elements. Pharmaceutical care is, however, provided for the direct benefit of the patient, and the pharmacist is responsible directly to the patient for the quality of that care. The fundamental relationship in pharmaceutical care is a mutually beneficial exchange in which the patient grants authority to the provider, and the provider gives competence and commitment (accepts responsibility) to the patient.

The fundamental goals, processes, and relationships of pharmaceutical care exist regardless of practice setting.

Source: Hepler CD, Strand LM. *Opportunities and responsibilities in pharmaceutical care*. Am J Pharm Educ. 1989;53(suppl):7S–15S.

Table 3.3 provides the definition of pharmaceutical care, as proposed by Hepler and Strand. Several trends are reflected in the concept. For many years, health care institutions and organizations had relied on process criteria in judging various systems. If a pharmacist used the correct process for filling and dispensing a prescription, then the results of that process were assumed to be of adequate quality. In the pharmaceutical care definition, contemporary outcome-oriented language is presented in the first paragraph. Thus, where a hospital in the past might have been required to have a certain type of drug distribution system, now the hospital would be checked for medication error rates. Instead of trying to define the process, only the outcomes were of interest.

For pharmaceutical care, the four outcomes as shown should be related to the purposes for which a medication is being administered to a patient, as defined in the first paragraph.

The team approach is endorsed in the second paragraph, reflecting pharmacy's shared purpose with other health care professions. Also identified in that paragraph are the kinds of functions a pharmacist would be expected to provide.

Covenant:
A promise or an agreement between two parties in which each provides something of value to the other. In pharmacy, the patient gives money to the pharmacist, who provides a patient-specific pharmaceutical product along with information on the proper use and adverse effects of that product.

The third paragraph is the key to the concept of pharmaceutical care. The pharmacist has a direct relationship with the patient and a direct responsibility to that patient to provide competent pharmaceutical care (as defined in the first two paragraphs). If the pharmacist was not providing services appropriate to those of a profession (value, complexity, and specificity), then Hepler argued that the pharmacist had broken his or her professional **covenant** with that patient.[3]

Finally, the fourth paragraph stated that the provision of pharmaceutical care should occur anytime and anywhere a pharmacist encountered a patient. Thus, the same principles applied whether the patient was in an intensive-care unit at a major medical center or was asking about a skin rash in a busy, **deep-discounting** chain or mass-merchandise pharmacy.

The concept of pharmaceutical care struck a responsive chord with many practitioners. It was termed pharmacy's mission for the 1990s,[6] and links between pharmaceutical care and the quality of care to patients were made.[7]

By 1990, the contributions that pharmacists could make clinically had been recognized by society through two key federal laws. In 1974 and again in 1987, the federal government ruled that consultant pharmacists must check the dose regimens of nursing home patients each month. In 1990, Congress passed a law that pharmacists must offer counsel to ambulatory Medicaid patients about these medications, and many state legislatures and boards of pharmacy extended this requirement to all patients through changes in pharmacy statutes and regulations.

The decision on the doctor of pharmacy degree

The pharmacy profession struggled and debated for 40 years as to what the appropriate entry-level degree for pharmacy should be. Finally, in the early 1990s, the profession settled on the doctor of pharmacy. But the battle took its toll on pharmacists and their national associations.

An increasing number of student pharmacists had been voluntarily seeking the PharmD degree during the 1980s, but many of them did so after first obtaining their baccalaureate degrees and, in many cases, working for a few years. Most pharmacy graduates (6,000 of 7,000 graduates in 1990), however, finished with BS degrees in pharmacy. By 1995, the enrollment in PharmD programs would total 9,346 individuals, compared with 24,069 in BS degree programs.

In 1932, the Accreditation Council for Pharmacy Education (ACPE) was founded as the national agency for the accreditation of professional degree programs in pharmacy and providers of continuing pharmacy education. In 1989, the ACPE announced plans to consider revising its accreditation standards to eliminate the BS Pharmacy degree by 2000. Because many state boards require pharmacists to be graduates of ACPE-approved programs, this ACPE action essentially eliminated the BS Pharmacy as an entry-level degree for pharmacy practice, replacing it with the PharmD credential.

By 1992, all major pharmacy practitioner organizations had endorsed a "new PharmD" as the entry-level degree. The course was affirmed that summer, when the House of Delegates of the American Association of Colleges of Pharmacy supported the PharmD as pharmacy's entry-level degree.

ACPE in 1997 finalized the standards for the PharmD programs of the twenty-first century, marking completion of nearly 10 years of hearings, confrontations, and oppositions about the profession's entry-level degree. Recently, ACPE released the 2016 *Accreditation Standards and Key Elements for the Professional Program in Pharmacy Leading to the Doctor of Pharmacy Degree.*[8] Today, all U.S. pharmacy schools offer only the PharmD as an entry credential for pharmacy practice.

In 2011, ACPE expanded its activities to include evaluation and certification of professional degree programs internationally. In 2014, ACPE collaborated with ASHP to accredit pharmacy technician education and training programs.

Deep discounter: A type of mercantile outlet that reduces prices far below those of normal retail outlets and relies on volume to make a profit.

Pharmaceutical care in community pharmacies and health systems

Until the mid-1990s, pharmaceutical care was provided primarily in hospitals with clinical pharmacy services and long-term-care facilities where consultant pharmacists reviewed medication therapy on a monthly basis. In community pharmacy, practice remained primarily as Hepler had described it: count, pour, lick, and stick.

In 1997, in the North Carolina mountain town of Asheville, that began to change. What became known as the Asheville Project was implemented when the city of Asheville tried to figure out how to contain its rapidly rising employee health costs. The result was a system in which pharmacists developed thriving pharmaceutical care practices in their local community pharmacies; employees, retirees, and dependents with diabetes had lower overall health costs, missed fewer days of work or school, and required less-intensive health care interventions; and the city found its health care dollars being spent to keep people well instead of dealing with their illnesses after they had worsened.[9-11] This positive experience with diabetes would be replicated in patients with asthma,[12] cardiovascular disease,[13] and depression (unpublished data).

As the Asheville Project got off the ground, William M. Ellis joined the APhA Foundation, and he brought a new level of energy to this venerable organization. The foundation's Quality Center initiated the Pinnacle Awards, given annually to recognize an individual, a group practice, health system, or corporation; and a government agency, nonprofit organization, or association to recognize pioneering, innovative ways to improve medication use processes that increase medication adherence, reduce drug misadventures, improve patient outcomes, and increase communication among all members of the health care team. The foundation sponsored Project ImPACT: Hyperlipidemia, a research study in which 26 pharmacies significantly improved serum cholesterol levels in 397 patients with dyslipidemias through education and adherence initiatives.[14] The Foundation also became involved in the Asheville Project including an effort to demonstrate the importance of patient self-management in diabetes,[15] a project that proved this local effort could be replicated in communities across the country in the Diabetes Ten City Challenge.[16]

As described further in Chapter 5, pharmacy achieved a ringing endorsement for the concept of pharmaceutical care in 2003 when the U.S. Congress created a medication therapy management (MTM) benefit as part of newly established prescription drug coverage (Part D) for the Medicare program, which covers the elderly and citizens with disabilities. The Medicare Prescription Drug, Improvement, and Modernization Act of 2003 required that MTM services be provided to high-risk patients with the goals of enhancing patients' understanding of appropriate drug use, increasing adherence to medication therapy, and improving the detection of adverse drug events.[17]

In keeping with the spirit and precepts of pharmaceutical care, MTM services go far beyond the brief counseling encounters required under the Omnibus Budget Reconciliation Act of 1990 (OBRA '90). A document presenting the consensus of national pharmacy organizations notes, "MTM services encompass the assessment and evaluation of the patient's complete medication therapy regimen, rather than focusing on an individual medication product. This model framework describes baseline core elements of MTM service delivery in pharmacy practice and does not represent all services that could be delivered by pharmacists."[17]

As presented in the second version of a "core elements" document, the MTM service model in pharmacy practice includes the following five core elements:[17]

- Medication therapy review
- Personal medication record
- Medication-related action plan
- Intervention and/or referral
- Documentation and follow-up

Similarly to the community setting, the *pharmaceutical care* term was embraced by the health care system associations. In 1992, the American Society of Health-System Pharmacists (ASHP) formally endorsed the concept.[18] ASHP defined the five principal elements of pharmaceutical care as follows:

- Medication related
- Care
- Outcomes
- Quality of life
- Responsibility

ASHP described *pharmaceutical care* as the *medication-related* care provided directly to patients to produce definite *outcomes*. These outcomes are intended to improve patients' *quality of life*, and the health care providers accept the *responsibility* for the patients' outcomes.

Patient care services: Expanding the role of pharmacists in public health

As pharmaceutical care led to significant advances for expanding pharmacists' role in various practice settings, a new term was used by APhA and other groups to encompass all pharmacist-provided services.

The term *patient care services* describes pharmacist-provided services across various health care settings. In the community setting, pharmacists help patients manage their self-care behaviors, improve continuity of care among health care providers, and enhance outcomes among patients with chronic diseases.

In integrated health care organizations, pharmacists coordinate the medication use process, provide disease management services, and optimize the use of resources. In addition, pharmacists provide medication-related expertise in interprofessional teams and contribute to continuous quality improvement initiatives in the organizations.

Recently, APhA released the 2016 *Pharmacists' Patient Care Services Digest*. Formerly known as the *APhA MTM Digest*, the scope of the publication was expanded to better reflect the expanded roles pharmacists are playing in public health.[19]

The Institute of Medicine (IOM) released several reports on the quality of health care services in the United States and education of health professionals. Overall, the IOM reports emphasized the need for redesigning the health care system and including interprofessional education in the training of health care providers.[20,21] The IOM reports resulted in key national and global educational reforms. The main goal of these initiatives

"Pharmacy has traditionally been an isolated profession; its ability to break out of its isolation will largely determine the success or otherwise of its public health role in the future."

—Stuart Anderson in Community pharmacy and public health in Great Britain, 1936 to 2006, J Epidemiol Community Health. 2007:61:844–8

is to better prepare health professionals to provide patient-centered care in high-performing interprofessional teams.

On the global level, two reports were published on the education of health professionals.[22,23] In 2010, the first global report was published by an independent commission on the education of health professionals indicated the needs to reform the education in medicine and other health care professions.[20] The World Health Organization (WHO) published the second report on interprofessional education.[23] This report provided a framework for defining and implementing interprofessional education. Specifically, the WHO defined interprofessional education as "students from two or more professions learning about, from, and with each other to enable effective collaborations and improve health outcomes."[23]

Based on the WHO framework, the Interprofessional Education Collaborative (IPEC) published its report *Core Competencies for Interprofessional Collaborative Practice*.[24] The 2011 report was sponsored by several professional health associations, including medicine, dentistry, pharmacy, nursing, and public health. The IPEC report specified the following four core domains of interprofessional education: values and ethics of interprofessional practice; roles and responsibilities; interprofessional communication; and teams and teamwork.

On the national level, ACPE mandated interprofessional education in the 2016 Standards and Key Elements for the Professional Program in Pharmacy Leading to the Doctor of Pharmacy Degree.[8] Building on the WHO and IPEC reports, ACPE adopted the core domains of interprofessional education for implementation in pharmacy curricula.[25]

According to the ACPE standard 3, pharmacy graduates must participate and actively engage as contributing health care team members by respecting and understanding the values of other professionals to better meet patients' needs.[8] Furthermore, standard 11 describes the following three key elements associated with interprofessional education.[8]

The first key element is interprofessional team dynamics. It highlights the need for student pharmacists to articulate the values and ethics of interprofessional practice sites, effectively communicate with other health professionals, and respect their roles and responsibilities. The second key element is interprofessional team education. It emphasizes that student pharmacists must contribute and advance the quality of patient care. In addition, the students must have opportunities to gain knowledge on the skills, abilities, and scope of practice of other team members.[8] The third key element is interprofessional team practice. It focuses on the importance that student pharmacists participate in experiential activities with prescribers and student-prescribers from other health care professions. Specifically, student pharmacists must be competent in providing direct patient care and participate in therapeutic decision making to enhance the effectiveness of the interprofessional care teams.[8]

Pharmacy: The future belongs to you

If they choose to be part of the solution to America's health care crisis, pharmacists are now positioned well to be the drug-therapy experts on the interprofessional health care team. The biotechnology and pharmacogenomics revolutions are producing complicated new drugs that defy categorization based on past schemes, and drugs are more important than ever in therapeutics. The bold decisions made about the critical role of pharmacists in public health have produced formal recognition of pharmacists' clinical services, including MTM and immunizations. Currently, many pharmacists are spending most of their time providing these services in their practice rather than in the drug preparation duties that dominated in the past.

REFERENCES

1. Hepler CD. Pharmacy as a clinical profession. *Am J Hosp Pharm*. 1985;42(6):1298–306.
2. Larsen MS. *The Rise of Professionalism*. Berkeley, Calif.: University of California Press; 1977.
3. Hepler CD. The third wave in pharmaceutical education: the clinical movement. *Am J Pharm Educ*. 1987;51(4):369–85.
4. Day RL, Goyan JE, Herfindal ET, Sorby DL. The origins of the clinical pharmacy program at the University of California, San Francisco. *DICP*. 1991;25(3):308–14.
5. Hepler CD, Strand LM. Opportunities and responsibilities in pharmaceutical care. *Am J Pharm Educ*. 1989;53(suppl):7S–15S.
6. Penna RP. Pharmaceutical care: pharmacy's mission for the 1990s. *Am J Hosp Pharm*. 1990;47(3):543–9.
7. Angaran DM. Quality assurance to quality improvement: measuring and monitoring pharmaceutical care. *Am J Hosp Pharm*. 1991;48(9):1901–7.
8. Accreditation Council for Pharmacy Education. *Accreditation Standards and Key Elements for the Professional Program in Pharmacy Leading to the Doctor of Pharmacy Degree ("Standards 2016")*. Chicago: Accreditation Council for Pharmacy Education; 2015.
9. Cranor CW, Christensen DB. The Asheville Project: short-term outcomes of a community pharmacy diabetes care program. *J Am Pharm Assoc*. 2003;43(2):149–59.
10. Cranor CW, Bunting BA, Christensen DB. The Asheville Project: long-term clinical and economic outcomes in a community pharmacy diabetes care program. *J Am Pharm Assoc*. 2003;43(2):173–84.
11. Garrett DG, Martin LA. The Asheville Project: participants' perceptions of factors contributing to the success of a Patient Self-Management Program for Diabetes. *J Am Pharm Assoc*. 2003;43(2):185–90.
12. Bunting BA, Cranor CW. The Asheville Project: long-term clinical, humanistic, and economic outcomes of a community-based medication therapy management program for asthma. *J Am Pharm Assoc*. 2006;46(2):133–47.
13. Bunting BA, Smith BH, Sutherland SE. The Asheville Project: Clinical and economic outcomes of a community-based long-term medication therapy management program for hypertension and dyslipidemia. *J Am Pharm Assoc*. 2008;48(1):23–31.
14. Bluml BM, McKenney JM, Cziraky MJ. Pharmaceutical care services and results in Project ImPACT: hyperlipidemia. *J Am Pharm Assoc*. 2000;40(2):157–65.
15. Garrett DG, Bluml BM. Patient self-management program for diabetes: first-year clinical, humanistic, and economic outcomes. *J Am Pharm Assoc*. 2005;45(2):130–7.
16. Fera T, Bluml BM, Ellis WM et al. The Diabetes Ten City Challenge: Interim clinical and humanistic outcomes of a multisite community pharmacy diabetes care program. *J Am Pharm Assoc*. 2008;48(2):181–90.
17. American Pharmacists Association, National Association of Chain Drug Stores Foundation, Bennett MS et al. Medication therapy management in pharmacy practice: core elements of an MTM service model (version 2.0). *J Am Pharm Assoc*. 2008;48(3):341–53.
18. Oddis JA. Report of the House of Delegates: June 1 and 3, 1992. *Am J Hosp Pharm*. 1992;49:1962–73.
19. American Pharmacists Association. *Pharmacists' Patient Care Services Digest: Building Momentum. Increasing Access*. Washington, D.C.: American Pharmacists Association; 2016. http://media.pharmacist.com/documents/APhA_Digest.pdf. Accessed March 29, 2016.

20. Institute of Medicine. *Preventing Medication Errors*. Washington, D.C.: National Academies Press; 2007.

21. Committee on Quality of Health Care in America, Institute of Medicine. *Crossing the Quality Chasm: A New Health Care System for the 21st Century*. Washington, D.C.: National Academy Press; 2001.

22. Frenk J, Chen L, Bhutta ZA et al. Health professionals for a new century: transforming education to strengthen health systems in an interdependent world. *Lancet*. 2010;376(9756):1923-58.

23. Health Professions Network Nursing & Midwifery Office, Human Resources for Health. *Framework for Action in Interprofessional Education and Collaborative Practice*. Geneva: World Health Organization; 2010. http://www.who.int/hrh/resources/framework_action/en/. Accessed March 9, 2016.

24. Interprofessional Education Collaborative Expert Panel. *Core Competencies for Interprofessional Collaborative Practice: Report of an Expert Panel*. Washington, D.C.: Interprofessional Education Collaborative; 2011. http://www.aacn.nche.edu/education-resources/ipecreport.pdf. Accessed March 10, 2016.

25. Kahaleh AA, Danielson J, Franson KL et al. An Interprofessional Education Panel on Development, Implementation, and Assessment Strategies. *Am J Pharm Educ*. 2015;79(6):78.

Chapter 4

Communications in Pharmacy Practice

Bruce A. Berger, PhD, RPh

Successful communication of information, ideas, and concepts is an important part of modern life, and it is an integral skill that must be learned, developed, and used by competent pharmacists. Medications are complicated technologies that must be used properly. Pharmacists can help patients make the best use of pharmacotherapy by making sure they understand the need for each drug, when and how to take it, and what benefits and adverse effects to expect.

For you, the new pharmacist in training, communication skills must be developed early in your studies. Direct patient contact is a component of early experiential programs in curricula of schools of pharmacy, and pharmacy students must be ready to talk with patients about their health and feelings. In addition, communication skills are important in group discussions and interdisciplinary projects used for teaching purposes within the school itself.

In this chapter, proven techniques that you can use to build relationships and improve patient care are described. This material is based on the third edition of a book published by APhA, *Communication Skills for Pharmacists: Building Relationships, Improving Patient Care*, by Bruce A. Berger, Emeritus Professor, Auburn University Harrison School of Pharmacy, and President, Berger Consulting, LLC. Further information about each topic is available in that text along with more complete lists of references. The textbook is available in print (pharmacist.com) and online at www.pharmacylibrary.com.

Developing the relationship

As described in Chapter 3, the concept of pharmaceutical care is based on a covenantal relationship between pharmacists and patients, and like all relationships, this one must be established and maintained. Without a patient-pharmacist relationship, pharmaceutical care and medication therapy management cannot be provided.

Relationships between patients and pharmacists are important for many reasons, but the key aspect for purposes of this chapter is that relationships provide the basis for effective and valued communications. Unless the pharmacist and patient know each other and recognize that the other is a living, breathing, feeling person—that is, unless they have a relationship—then it is all too easy to simply view the other party as an impediment or nuisance who keeps us from doing what we really want to do.

Learning Objectives

Upon completion of this chapter, the reader should be able to:

1. Define and discuss the importance of the pharmacist–patient relationship in the context of communications.

2. Name the elements involved in active listening and empathic responding.

3. Describe the importance of supportive communication in pharmacists' interactions with patients.

4. Define and describe patient counseling.

5. Describe a process for communicating with physicians.

6. Differentiate between immediate and nonimmediate communications and describe how the amount of immediate language can be increased.

Acknowledgment: Content of this chapter is based on Bruce A. Berger's *Communication Skills for Pharmacists: Building Relationships, Improving Patient Care*, third edition, published by the American Pharmacists Association. Many of its ideas, examples, and concepts appeared originally in *U.S. Pharmacist* and were adapted with permission of Jobson Medical Information LLC, publisher of that journal.

Chapter 4

"Can I permit myself to enter into the private world of my patients, explore their feelings without judging them, and in some significant and honest way, respond in a manner that lets them know that I have listened and I want to provide whatever assistance or comfort that I can? Can I see this person as unique in his/her reaction to illness? Can I see what is different and the same about this person so that any insight or assistance I may give is the most useful to this patient?"

—Bruce A. Berger

Objectification:
The viewing of other people in a self-centered way, such as obstacles to one's own goals or a vehicle through which one's own goals can be realized without regard for the feelings of the other person.

In books published by the Arbinger Institute, two ways of responding to people are described: the responsive way and the resistant way.[1,2] When we recognize that other people are complex human beings with feelings, wants, and dreams, we treat them *responsively*. We appreciate their successes and their joys, and we respond to those feelings. But when we deal with other people in the *resistant way*, we treat them as vehicles, obstacles, or irrelevant (**objectification**), and our own self-centeredness prevents us from recognizing their human qualities. Such an attitude impairs or impedes the proper provision of information needed as part of the process of pharmaceutical care.[3,4]

The term *mental health* means "happiness" for many people, but a more correct definition for it is the adjustment of one's internal tensions rather than attempts to change the external environment to fit our own selfish wants. As pointed out by Peck in his classic 1978 book, *The Road Less Traveled*,[5] the first great realization of the Buddha was that life is suffering, resulting in disease and old age, and that in fact these are inevitable outcomes of life as we know it. As people recognize that they daily face a certain degree of suffering and learn ways of coping with it, they achieve mental health in the sense I have described here.

In pharmacy, we often encounter our patients at times when they have just learned that they have an acute or chronic disease or after they have found out that they have cancer or some other terminal condition. During the course of a busy day in the pharmacy or a frustrating time in our own lives, we must remember the nature of the covenant we have with our patients. As patients struggle to balance their own feelings with the realities of their lives, we as pharmacists should remember a few basic tenets that underlie healthy responses in such situations.

First, people behave in certain ways to get their needs met. In the pharmacy, patients may complain because it is the only way they know to get attention. They may be dealing with stress and have only dysfunctional strategies for dealing with change, loss, or disappointment. But somewhere underlying behaviors are feelings, and the pharmacist's recognition of those emotional needs may provide much information about how to best help patients with their medications and diseases.

Second, feelings are real. Feelings provide us with feedback—be they physical sensations such as heat or pain or the emotional feelings of joy, happiness, or loss. Feelings come from within one's self; they are not caused by other people. Feelings are caused by those meanings we assign others' communications in a given context. As health professionals, we are expected to appropriately manage our own feelings even as we acknowledge and validate the feelings of our patients. This can be difficult. We must remember that we can be aware of our own feelings and our rights to feel that way, but we should not inappropriately express those feelings to our patients.

Third, patients ultimately have responsibility for their own medication-taking behaviors, but we can have substantial influence over those behaviors. As pharmacists, we promise to provide patients with the medications they need, the information necessary for proper use of those medications, and the monitoring needed to safeguard patients' health during the medication use process. Patients pay us for these services. Although we cannot be held responsible for solving patients' problems, we can provide them with the best tools available for addressing those concerns and create an environment in which effective communication can occur. Although ultimately patients must take responsibility for taking medicines when and how they should, we play a major role in assisting them with this by providing thorough and accurate information and taking time to answer their questions and address their concerns.

Fourth, communication can be evaluated as appropriate or inappropriate only in relation to the objectives of the communicator. As pharmacists, we are in control of our own communication goals, and we should strive to keep those professional and appropriate to the mission of improving patients' health.

Finally, unrealistic expectations can drive you crazy. Pharmacists are quite familiar with the patient who constantly complains about medication prices. Yet because these individuals return month after month to make purchases, and they apparently feel the need to complain, they obviously are more than willing to buy the pharmacy's products and services at the fair price offered. Remember, life is suffering, and the fact that patients complain may be more related to that than to any of their specific complaints.

Listening and empathic responding

To demonstrate the depth and meaning of the professional relationship with a patient, the pharmacist must hear, understand, and respond effectively to the concerns expressed by the patient. To do so requires a great deal of active effort and, in a sense, courage. Let me explain.

Listening begins with an act of will; we must choose to listen—really listen—to someone else (Figure 4.1). Active listening requires our complete and undivided attention. By giving our patients our attention and focusing our energies upon them, we show each patient that we have a trusting, caring relationship, one embodied in the concept of pharmaceutical care.

Figure 4.1 | The process of listening and empathic response.

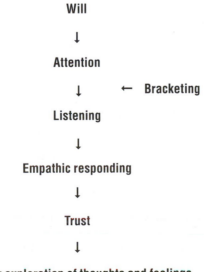

Will

↓

Attention

↓   ← Bracketing

Listening

↓

Empathic responding

↓

Trust

↓

Further exploration of thoughts and feelings

True listening requires the listener to temporarily suspend his or her own beliefs, opinions, and ideas, a process called *bracketing* by psychologists.[5] The greatest barrier to this type of listening is our tendency to judge or evaluate the information using our own ideals. When we do so, we have not listened, and we simply lump the patient into a stereotyped category and fail to truly understand the unique emotions the patient has about a newly diagnosed chronic or terminal disease, the fear of being pregnant after a birth control method failed, or an unexpected adverse effect of a medication. Great courage is required to truly listen, because when we suspend our values, we open ourselves to the chance that we may need to change our own ideas or beliefs.

After we truly listen to patients, our next responsibility as pharmacists is to respond empathically. Empathy is different from sympathy, which is one's own emotional response to the problems of another. Empathy is the feeling or experiencing of another's affective response to a problem or situation. As with true listening, this experiencing is done without the interference of one's own values or judgments. Although many people think they can be more empathic if they have personally experienced a similar loss or tragedy, that is not necessarily the case, because one's own emotional perspective about the situation may get in the way of seeing the patient's unique perspective.

When pharmacists respond with empathy to our patients, we show courage, because the process requires the opening up of one's self to the pain and other affective responses that people have to the problems in their lives. Thus, empathy is often not all soothing—in fact, it can be quite painful and unsettling.

In many situations we find ourselves in as pharmacists, we must remember that empathy does not mean that we have to give up our own values, ideals, opinions, or positions. We can express our understanding of others' situations without unauthorized (and illegal) dispensing of prescription drugs or controlled substances, loaning money to employees or patients, or placing orders from sales representatives for goods we do not need.

Finally, remember that we must respond empathically for patients to know that we care about them and their health problems. The best way to do this is to reflect back what patients are saying to us. We should not minimize the problem, try to claim that the patient has nothing to worry about, or maintain that the patient should not be so depressed. Whatever emotions or difficulties the patient expresses as we truly listen, those should be reflected back to demonstrate an empathic response.

Supportive communication

Many of the patient–pharmacist interactions described in this chapter have involved situations in which patients were upset or concerned about their health status. Pharmacists commonly encounter patients with such apprehensions, and as a result, they often need to engage in supportive communication.

Supportive communication allows people to feel understood and less alone.[6] When patients express their concerns openly and physicians respond to them, studies have shown that patient **adherence** to therapy is greater, health professionals are more satisfied with the relationship, and patients perceive their physicians to be more understanding

Adherence:
The rate at which patients actually take a prescribed treatment. Known formerly as *compliance*. A related term, *persistence*, describes the rate at which patients continue to take their medications over time.

and caring.[7] A study of physician interactions with patients showed that supportive communication had physical and health benefits, improved resistance to infection and disease, and even extended life.[8]

Pharmacists can be supportive in their communications by legitimizing the patient's feelings, acknowledging the importance and permanence of the loss to the patient, and encouraging the patient to accept the loss.[7] These losses can involve loss of mobility or independence, or of habits the patient considers good, desirable, or pleasurable, such as certain foods or smoking.

In validating the patient's feelings, we as pharmacists can use the processes and techniques described above under listening and empathic responses. When we do, we must remember that our goal is to demonstrate caring and concern for the patient so the patient is better prepared to deal with the anger and fear he or she may be feeling, accept his or her situation, and be more likely to adhere to treatments.

The goal of supportive communication is not to solve the patient's problems, to cheer the patient up, or make everything better. No matter what we say or do, the patient may remain upset or agitated. Consider this situation: a patient storms into the pharmacy, demanding that a prescription be filled immediately because the person has a flight to catch. You are busy, with several patients who have waited 20 minutes or more for their medications. In this situation, you must communicate supportively with the patient, but you should not accept responsibility for the patient's failure to plan ahead. It will take a certain amount of uninterrupted time to convey to this patient that you understand his problem but that you also have responsibilities to other patients. But the alternative is more costly.

When patients have diseases or conditions that evoke shame or feelings of guilt, they often convert these emotions to anger, and pharmacists may sometimes bear the brunt of their frustration. The stigma society attaches to conditions such as depression or HIV infection makes patients' feelings understandable, and pharmacists should make every effort to communicate with these patients in a supportive manner and to avoid responding to their anger with attacks or avoidance. More than most, these patients need support and confirmation.

In dealing with patients who are upset, we should avoid conveying unhelpful or unsupportive messages, including ones that show that we are trying to fix the problem. We must learn to simply listen and legitimize feelings, for that is what will alleviate some of these people's stress.

Patient counseling

As you advance in pharmacy school, you will increasingly be called upon to provide information to patients about their medications and the diseases being treated. This will happen initially in your early pharmacy practice experiences, but you may also find that, in social situations or at family reunions, people will ask you questions about their own experiences with medications. Later, during advanced pharmacy practice experiences and courses in which you deal directly with patients, you—as the emerging drug therapy expert on the health care team—will apply your unique knowledge and skills in helping patients understand how to best use their medications in the prevention and treatment of disease.

Patient counseling is the general term for provision of information to patients in such settings. Required by law (see Chapter 7), patient counseling should accompany the dispensing of every prescription. However, here we refer to patient counseling as an *exchange* of information. We give information about the patient's medicines and condition, but we also get information about what the patient already knows and what concerns may exist (see Table 4.1). It is not enough to coerce patients into signing away their right to counseling as part of the transfer of medications by pharmacy staff, as is done far too often in many of the nation's community pharmacies. The pharmacist is a professional with responsibilities to the patient that are required under law, regulation, and the profession's own code of ethics (see Chapter 5), and the privilege of being a pharmacist can be revoked if the person does not comply with these requirements. Along with getting the right drug to the right patient at the right time, the provision of adequate information about the medication is a basic responsibility that we have as pharmacists.

The scope and nature of patient counseling will become clearer as you advance in the curriculum of your school of pharmacy. For now, consider the steps in the checklist shown in Table 4.1, and begin thinking about how you will convey in simple terms the information you are beginning to learn about medications.

Interacting with physicians

Another situation you may soon experience is interacting on a professional level with physicians. Although pharmacists often contact physicians about potential errors made in the prescribing process, a collaborative relationship must be established between these members of the health care team. Out of mutual concern over the best interests of the patient, pharmacists and physicians must develop mutual respect for one another.

As a pharmacist in training, you will mostly be in situations where you are a temporary member of a health care unit. But as you enter practice, you will be in more permanent situations, and in these it is important to begin building rapport with your physician colleagues before you need to contact them about a specific patient. A pharmacy's innovative services can be presented in one-on-one meetings with physicians or through lectures to local medical societies. Volunteering to work on public health or disaster-preparedness committees in your community is another forum within which to interact with physicians and other health care professionals. In each of these efforts, one goal is to establish yourself as a professional with a unique set of knowledge and skills that are of value to the other members of the health care team and to the community.

Drug interactions:
Detrimental (or occasionally positive) effects produced when two or more drugs are used at the same time. By checking the patient profile for interacting drugs, the computer can alert the pharmacist to consider whether both drugs can be safely used together in a patient.

When situations arise in which the pharmacist needs to call a physician, the focus of that communication should be on the patient and drug-related problems that need to be solved or averted. These may involve **drug interactions**, diseases that have not been recognized or treated, suboptimal medication choice, or incorrect dosages. Whatever the problem, the pharmacist should be prepared before contacting the physician, including having a recommendation and a rationale for that solution to the problem.

During a face-to-face encounter or a telephone call, follow this process for communicating with the physician and his or her staff:

Table 4.1 | Patient Counseling Checklist

1. Introduces self.
2. Identifies patient or patient's agent.
3. Asks if patient has time to discuss medication.
4. Explains purpose and importance of counseling session.
5. Asks patient what physician told him or her about medication and what it is treating. Asks what patient knows or understands about the disease. Uses any available patient profile information (including possible allergies).
6. Asks patient if he or she has any concerns prior to information provision.
7. Responds with appropriate empathy, listening, and attention to concerns. Uses these skills throughout counseling session.
8. Tells patient name, indication, and route of administration of the medication.
9. Tells patient the dosage regimen.
10. Asks patient if he or she will have a problem taking the medication as prescribed.
11. Tailors medication regimen to patient's daily routine.
12. Tells patient how long it will take for the medication to show an effect.
13. Tells patient how long he or she might be on the medication.
14. Tells patient when he or she is due back for a refill (and number of refills).
15. Emphasizes the benefits of the medication and supports its use before talking about side effects and barriers.
16. Discusses major side effects of the drug and whether they will go away in time.
17. Points out that additional rare (emphasizes this to patient) side effects are listed in the information sheet (to be given to patient at the end of counseling session). Encourages patient to call if he or she has any concerns about these.
18. Uses written information to support counseling where appropriate.
19. Discusses precautions (e.g., activities to avoid).
20. Discusses beneficial activities (e.g., exercise, decreased salt intake, diet, self-monitoring).
21. Discusses drug–drug, drug–food, and drug–disease interactions.
22. Discusses storage recommendations and ancillary instructions (e.g., shake well, refrigerate).
23. Explains to patient in precise terms what to do if he or she misses a dose.
24. Checks for understanding by asking patient to repeat back key information (e.g., drug name, side effects, what to do about missed doses).
25. Rechecks for any additional concerns or questions.
26. Advises patients to always check their medicines before they leave the pharmacy.
27. Uses appropriate language throughout counseling session.
28. Maintains control of counseling session.
29. Organizes information in an appropriate manner.
30. Follows up to determine how patient is doing.

Source: Developed by the author of this chapter and Bill G. Felkey, a faculty colleague at the Auburn University Harrison School of Pharmacy. Reprinted from Berger BA. *Communication Skills for Pharmacists: Building Relationships, Improving Patient Care*, 3rd ed. Washington, D.C.: American Pharmacists Association; 2009.

---

1. State who you are and the purpose of the call. Be pleasant: "Hello, Dr. Jones. I am Joe Smith from Smith's Pharmacy. I need to talk with you about Carla Brown's prescription for (name of medication). Is this a good time?"
2. State the problem and recommended solution: "You prescribed (name of prescribed medication) for Carla. She does not have any third-party coverage and would have to pay for this medication out of her own pocket. She says she cannot afford it. I would like to recommend (name of alternative medication) if you are treating (indication). This would be affordable to her and would be equally or nearly as effective."
3. If you meet resistance: Stay focused on the problem. Make good eye contact (if in person), and repeat back your understanding of what the physician's resistance is about. "So, if I understand you correctly, you simply don't like (name of alternative medication) because you have had better success with (name of prescribed medication)." The physician confirms this, and you state, "Given that you are treating (indication), I have found (give citation of study), and it shows that (name of alternative

medication) is very effective. I'm very concerned that Ms. Brown won't take the (name of prescribed medication) because it is too expensive for her. I have tried to convince her that it might prevent future visits, but she insists that she won't take it. Can we try (name of alternative medication) instead?"

Professional communications of this nature do much to establish, maintain, and strengthen the collegial relationship between pharmacists and physicians who work together in caring for patients. By focusing on the problem, relying on facts, and staying away from interpersonal conflicts, these health care professionals provide the best possible care for their patients.

Immediacy: Word choice and nonverbal cues

Much of the discussion in this chapter has focused on the central messages that you as a pharmacist in training should convey to patients and colleagues in various situations. But those messages are only a small part of the communication process—7% in some studies. The message received is influenced more by how you say something and what your body does while you are saying it. About 55% of the meaning attached to communications comes from nonverbal clues, and the other 38% comes from vocal cues.[9]

The choice of words used in a communication is important. For instance, the difference between saying "you and I should discuss this matter" and "we should discuss this matter" is great. The sentences technically mean the same thing, but use of "we" implies much greater verbal immediacy and greater sense of unity in solving a problem.

What is nonimmediate language? Consider the differences in perceived meaning by the following statements that all convey the same information:
• Remember, we said that you should come in for a checkup. (most immediate)
• Remember, you said that you would come in for a checkup.
• Remember, it was said that you should come in for a checkup. (least immediate)

Nonimmediate language is used by both patients and professionals to discuss topics with which they are uncomfortable, including death, dying, and serious conditions such as AIDS. Such distancing behavior is a normal means of coping with uncomfortable subjects or possibilities, but it fails to help patients address and accept their situations.

A three-step process can be used to increase the amount of immediate language in your communications:
1a. Identify topics and issues that make you uncomfortable, and
1b. Identify groups and persons with whom you feel uncomfortable.
2. Identify nonimmediate language when it is spoken.
3. Identify when and with whom you use nonimmediate language.

By recognizing when and how we are switching from open, direct language to words that create distance and discomfort, we are taking the first step toward improving our ability to convey empathy and provide truly supportive communications.

Nonverbal cues in communications come from a variety of indicators:

- How far away we stand while talking with others (proxemics)
- Use of time in our communications (chronemics)
- Amount of eye contact or gaze (oculesics)
- Use of touch (haptics)
- Body movements (kinesics)
- Use and choice of objects in communications, such as clothing and symbols (objectics)
- Use and quality of the voice, such as changes in tone and pitch (vocalics)

Nonverbal means of communication are very important in our discussions with patients. If we show boredom or disregard in our facial expressions, patients will believe those messages and ignore noncongruent words and messages. Windows and counters in prescription departments and elevation of pharmacists above the patients create barriers to effective communication. Americans are resentful when they are made to wait for more than 5 minutes in most situations.[10] Eye contact is very important in communicating understanding and caring. Touching a patient's arm can be an effective means of conveying empathy if the health professional does so in a comfortable and appropriate manner. All of these elements must be incorporated into the pharmacist's professional demeanor so that patients comprehend conveyed communications correctly and perceive that their pharmacist is a trusting, caring professional with whom a strong relationship is paramount.

Conclusion

The ability to communicate is important for every pharmacist. By beginning to develop the skills described in this chapter, you will be ready when the time comes for you to convey important information about medications with your family, your friends, and your patients.

References

1. Arbinger Institute. *Leadership and Self-Deception: Getting Out of the Box.* San Francisco: Barrett-Koehler Publishers; 2002.
2. Warner CT. *Bonds That Make Us Free: Healing Our Relationships, Coming to Ourselves.* Salt Lake City: Deseret Book Company; 2001.
3. Berger BA, Smith RE. Patient interaction. Part 1. The right choice. *US Pharm.* 2003(Apr).
4. Smith RE, Berger BA. The right choice: a pharmacy fable. Part 2. *US Pharm.* 2003(May).
5. Peck MS. *The Road Less Traveled.* New York: Simon & Schuster; 1978.
6. Basch MF. Empathic understanding: a review of the concept and some theoretical considerations. *J Am Psychoanal Assoc.* 1983;31:101–6.
7. Squier RW. A model of empathic understanding and adherence to treatment regimens in practitioner–patient relationships. *Soc Sci Med.* 1990;30:325–39.
8. Albrecht TL, Burleson BR, Goldsmith D. Supportive communication. In: Knapp ML, Miller GR, eds. *Handbook of Interpersonal Communication.* 2nd ed. Thousand Oaks, Calif.: Sage Publications; 1994.
9. Mehrabian A. *Silent Messages.* Belmont, Calif.: Wadsworth Publishing; 1971.
10. McCroskey JC. *An Introduction to Rhetorical Communication.* Englewood Cliffs, N.J.: Prentice Hall; 1982.

Chapter 5 | Ethics in Pharmacy Practice

L. Michael Posey

In Chapters 3 and 4, reference was made to the idea of a covenant, or promise, between the pharmacist and the patient. This professional covenant is similar to a legal contract, in which each party makes certain promises. In this case, the pharmacist agrees to provide pharmaceutical care to the patient, and the patient agrees to provide payment and any needed information to the pharmacist.

Implicit in this covenant is the idea that the pharmacist has certain moral obligations to the patient, specifically to provide quality pharmaceutical care. A component of pharmaceutical care is the provision of drug therapy that will improve the patient's health or well-being. What happens if the patient doesn't want to take the drug, even though the pharmacist knows the patient may suffer or even die as a result? What if the patient needs the drug but has no money to pay the pharmacist for it? What if the pharmacist knows that the patient is an alcoholic and an alternative drug is available that doesn't interact with alcohol? What if the drug is for AIDS and the pharmacist knows that the patient's wife is unaware of her husband's condition?

Each of these situations represents an ethical dilemma requiring choices that the pharmacist must make. Because of their professional roles, pharmacists have access to, or knowledge of, confidential information. Patients turn to pharmacists as knowledgeable, competent advisors about drug therapy and health care in general, and they expect to deal with an ethical, competent practitioner.

While much has been written about some of the major controversial ethical issues of our day—decisions about death and dying (assisted suicide, abortion), about rationing of health care resources, about who should make health care decisions (payers, patients, or health care providers)—pharmacists often encounter the simplest but most irreconcilable problems. A prominent citizen may ask for an unauthorized but medically needed refill on a Saturday when the prescribing physician is unavailable. A local physician may be overprescribing diet pills, but the pharmacy may be making a lot of money filling these questionable prescriptions. A physician may prescribe a **placebo** or nonprescription drug for a **hypochondriac** and ask the pharmacist to counsel the patient as if the medicine were a powerful analgesic. In social settings, pharmacists and student pharmacists are often asked about the usual use of certain medicines, whether a medication can cause a certain effect, and whether a given dose is "a lot".

In these and many other situations, pharmacists must make ethical decisions every day. Health care professionals have struggled with some of these situations since the days when the Hippocratic Oath was written; other dilemmas are the result of modern technologies that can preserve people as legally alive but mentally deceased. But what is ethics? What are the ethical principles that pharmacists can use as guides in making these difficult decisions?

Learning Objectives

Upon completion of this chapter, the reader should be able to:

1. Describe the moralistic basis of biomedical ethics.

2. Differentiate among ethical theories, principles, rules, and particular judgments and actions.

3. Compare and contrast the principles of beneficence and nonmaleficence.

4. Define and give pharmacy-specific examples of the principles of respect for patient autonomy, nonmaleficence, beneficence, and justice.

"As to disease, make a habit of two things — to help, or at least to do no harm."

—Hippocratic Oath

Placebo:
A preparation with no known pharmacologic or medicinal properties. Placebos can sometimes "work" by making the patient believe that a real drug is being given, and placebos are used in some research as a way of identifying the beneficial properties of drugs.

Hypochondriac:
A patient with a psychological disorder in which he or she complains of imagined medical problems.

The moralistic basis of biomedical ethics

In all human societies in the world, various behaviors are deemed to be right or wrong based on moralistic codes; these behaviors can be very different from culture to culture. In one of the best textbooks on biomedical ethics, Beauchamp and Childress differentiate between general moral codes, which apply to all members of a society, and professional moral codes, which apply to groups of people engaged in a certain profession or occupation.[1]

Beauchamp and Childress use the following logic sequence to illustrate four hierarchies of moral reasoning:

4. *Ethical theories* are derived from
3. *Principles*, which are derived from
2. *Rules*, which are derived from
1. *Particular judgments and actions*

As these levels suggest, people first learn about moral reasoning as small children by observing their own and others' actions and developing opinions about right and wrong. These opinions are codified into rules, which kindergarten and elementary school children use in a strict "good versus bad" view of the world. As a child matures, he or she develops principles of behavior that can be used as guides in the moralistic dilemmas of adolescence. And finally, ethical theories are developed by an individual, a group of individuals, or society as a whole (through the laws and court system) to guide behavior when rules and principles may conflict with one another.

Within pharmacy, moralistic reasoning is embodied in various professional codes of conduct. The most universal in the profession is that of the American Pharmacists Association (Table 5.1). Of the two major schools of thought in Western ethics, the APhA Code tends to take the position of the nonconsequentialists, which is based on the following principles:[2]

1. Autonomy: An action is right if it respects the autonomy, or independent choice, of others.
2. Veracity: Telling the truth is right.
3. Fidelity: Keeping promises, commitments, contracts, and covenants is right.
4. Avoiding killing: Taking of human life is wrong.
5. Justice: Fair distribution of goods and harms is right.

The other major school of thought, consequentialism, generally considers actions to be right when they have beneficial outcomes for the people involved and wrong if they have detrimental consequences. This line of reasoning is embodied in the principle of beneficence, which is a person's moral obligation to help others—to contribute to the welfare of others. Beneficence may be thought of as the Good Samaritan, a person who interrupts his or her own life so that a person in need can be assisted. The principle of nonmaleficence is somewhat different from this concept: The health care professional should above all keep the patient from harm.[2] These two principles are embodied in this quote from the Hippocratic Oath: "As to disease, make a habit of two things—to help, or at least to do no harm."

When discussing ethical issues in a chapter as brief as this one, it is difficult to maintain a separation between beneficence and nonmaleficence. In medicine, as in the world

Table 5.1. | Code of Ethics of the American Pharmacists Association[a]

Preamble: Pharmacists are health professionals who assist individuals in making the best use of medications. This Code, prepared and supported by pharmacists, is intended to state publicly the principles that form the fundamental basis of the roles and responsibilities of pharmacists. These principles, based on moral obligations and virtues, are established to guide pharmacists in relationships with patients, health professionals, and society.

I. A pharmacist respects the covenantal relationship between the patient and pharmacist.

Considering the patient–pharmacist relationship as a covenant means that a pharmacist has moral obligations in response to the gift of trust received from society. In return for this gift, a pharmacist promises to help individuals achieve optimum benefit from their medications, to be committed to their welfare, and to maintain their trust.

II. A pharmacist promotes the good of every patient in a caring, compassionate, and confidential manner.

A pharmacist places concern for the well-being of the patient at the center of professional practice. In doing so, a pharmacist considers needs stated by the patient as well as those defined by health science. A pharmacist is dedicated to protecting the dignity of the patient. With a caring attitude and a compassionate spirit, a pharmacist focuses on serving the patient in a private and confidential manner.

III. A pharmacist respects the autonomy and dignity of each patient.

A pharmacist promotes the right of self-determination and recognizes individual self-worth by encouraging patients to participate in decisions about their health. A pharmacist communicates with patients in terms that are understandable. In all cases, a pharmacist respects personal and cultural differences among patients.

IV. A pharmacist acts with honesty and integrity in professional relationships.

A pharmacist has a duty to tell the truth and to act with conviction of conscience. A pharmacist avoids discriminatory practices, behavior or work conditions that impair professional judgment, and actions that compromise dedication to the best interests of patients.

V. A pharmacist maintains professional competence.

A pharmacist has a duty to maintain knowledge and abilities as new medications, devices, and technologies become available and as health information advances.

VI. A pharmacist respects the values and abilities of colleagues and other health professionals.

When appropriate, a pharmacist asks for the consultation of colleagues or other health professionals or refers the patient. A pharmacist acknowledges that colleagues and other health professionals may differ in the beliefs and values they apply to the care of the patient.

VII. A pharmacist serves individual, community, and societal needs.

The primary obligation of a pharmacist is to individual patients. However, the obligations of a pharmacist may at times extend beyond the individual to the community and society. In these situations, the pharmacist recognizes the responsibilities that accompany these obligations and acts accordingly.

VIII. A pharmacist seeks justice in the distribution of health resources.

When health resources are allocated, a pharmacist is fair and equitable, balancing the needs of patients and society.

[a] Adopted by the membership of the American Pharmaceutical (now Pharmacists) Association, October 27, 1994.

in general, no action or procedure is completely safe or completely effective. Thus, the line can blur between doing good and not doing harm, for in doing good one can inadvertently do harm. However, it is important to differentiate between the two concepts so that ethical dilemmas may be properly analyzed.

Medical ethics is derived from a combination of the above elements, but the subject can be discussed by looking at four principles that embody all of the above concepts:
- Respect for patient autonomy
- Nonmaleficence
- Beneficence
- Justice

From these four principles come the obligations of the professional to be truthful with patients (veracity), to respect a patient's wishes to be left alone (privacy), to not disclose without permission information about the patient's medical condition (confidentiality), and to keep promises made to the patient (fidelity). Let's look at each of these underlying principles in more detail.

Respect for autonomy

In medicine, the principle of respect for autonomy is manifest in various types of informed consent to treatment and medical research. Medicine at one time operated under a paternalistic system in which the physician was considered the best decision maker, since he or she had the range of knowledge about the disease state, the available alternatives, and the patient's condition. However, people have now realized that the risk-benefit ratio for a medical intervention is often quite different when considered by a patient whose life might be endangered by the procedure and a physician who stands to gain materially if the procedure is performed. This conflict has now been largely resolved by acceptance of the principle of respect for autonomy into medical practice: It is the patient who makes the final decision about whether a procedure will be performed on his or her body.

Five elements of informed consent must be met for the patient to make a proper decision about whether to submit to certain medical treatments:[1]
I. Threshold element
    A. Competence
II. Information elements
    A. Disclosure of information
    B. Understanding of information
III. Consent elements
    A. Voluntariness
    B. Authorization

Competence refers to the ability of the patient to understand the decision at hand. Comatose patients cannot communicate and therefore are unable to provide informed consent. Other types of physical incompetence may also prevent informed decisions, as can cases of psychological incompetence (for example, patients with Alzheimer's disease or memory impairment).

In such cases, the next of kin or legal guardian of the patient must make an informed decision about therapy. Many life-or-death decisions end up in court when the decision of the legal guardian or relatives conflicts with institutional policies, laws, or other people's opinions. People are increasingly preparing documents known as living wills, or advance directives, that attempt to spell out in advance what decisions they would make in certain clinical situations. Or patients may sign a durable power of attorney for health care, which allows spouses or other persons who know the patients well to make such decisions in cases of incompetence.

Whatever the situation, informed consent or refusal of treatment cannot occur without either a competent patient or a legal guardian involved.

The informational elements include both disclosure and understanding. Disclosure must be appropriate based on contemporary professional standards or appropriate for what a "reasonable person" would expect to be told in a similar situation. Exceptions to the disclosure element have been recognized in cases of emergency or when "sound medical judgment" would lead the health care professional to not disclose certain information to, for example, a depressed or an unstable patient.[1]

Assuring that the patient understands the decision being made is quite problematic, since the means to measure understanding are often unavailable. Some patients are capable of understanding one day but not the next. Others may be in a stage of denial about their disease and thereby be incapable of understanding the relevance of a medical procedure. Patients' definitions of medical terms may vary substantially, thus impeding understanding. Or a procedure may be explained only minutes before it is to occur, giving the patient insufficient time to process the information before a decision is required.[1]

Because of the wide variability of problems with understanding as an element of informed consent, no clearly established models or definitions exist. But health professionals continue to have an ethical obligation to assure that patients truly understand the options they have when making informed decisions about their medical care.

Finally, the patient must give consent voluntarily and authorize a procedure through a legally valid document. *Voluntariness*, as used here, is defined this way: "A person acts voluntarily to the degree he or she wills the action without being under the control of another agent's influence."[1] Thus, voluntariness can be affected by coercion or manipulation by health professionals or relatives and by drugs or psychological disorders. Manipulation is the presentation of information in such a way that the patient's view of the situation is altered so that the patient does what the manipulator wants.

Thus, the patient has the right under currently held ethical principles to make autonomous decisions, and health care professionals should respect them. This should be not confused with autonomy itself, but rather it is restricted to a respect for autonomous decision making. However, this is but one element underlying biomedical ethical principles, and it must be considered along with the other three elements: nonmaleficence, beneficence, and justice.[1]

Nonmaleficence

Nonmaleficence is best summarized in the most famous sentence in the Hippocratic Oath: "At least, do no harm." It is differentiated from beneficence in that nonmaleficence refers to not taking actions that would inflict harm, whereas beneficence refers to taking actions that will do good. Conflict between the two principles is inevitable, since no medical or drug treatment is completely effective or completely safe; there are always cases of therapeutic failure and adverse unintended consequences.

Negligence:
Failure of a professional to provide the standard of due care to patients who seek that care.

The principle of nonmaleficence is integrated into a professional standard of due care, which is the basis used by courts in trying professional misconduct or **negligence** cases. The moralistic due care standard, comprising the following elements, is similar to the legalistic standard of due care:[1]
- The professional must have a duty to the affected party.
- The professional must breach that duty.
- The affected party must experience harm or injury.
- This harm must be caused by the breach of duty.

All four elements must be met; if the professional is not recognized by society or the courts as having a duty to a specific patient, then no breach has occurred. Similarly, if the patient does not experience harm or if the harm does not result from the breach of duty, no breach is recognized.

Over the past two decades, several widely publicized court cases have involved conflicts over the principle of nonmaleficence, often in situations that require a distinction between allowing a patient to die versus killing a patient. Generally recognized is that health care professionals should provide due care to patients but are not obligated to provide care, especially "heroic" means, when biological death is imminent in a person with serious or severe illnesses or conditions. The range of pertinent distinctions is as follows:[1]

I. Obligatory care
II. Optional care (may be neutral or heroic care)
III. Wrong care (obligatory not to provide)

Living will:
A legal document that provides guidance to healthcare professionals about what actions a patient would like taken if he or she is unable to provide an informed decision because of illness or injury. Also known as an advance directive.

How does a medical professional decide what care should be provided to a given patient? Three factors are involved: the patient's clinical condition, the patient's prior wishes as expressed informally or in a **living will**, and laws and societal rules.

Courts have generally supported the withholding of care—including such basic needs as nutrition and respiratory support—to patients whose mental function is minimal or nonexistent and whose conditions are considered irreversible. In cases where no living will is available, the next of kin, legal guardian, or designated proxy is consulted about the possible courses of action. Thus, even obligatory care may not be necessary in every patient care situation.

Heroic measures are a result of modern scientific and technological developments that provide people with ways of prolonging life even though a person is clinically nonfunctional. For example, in nursing homes, the acceptability of failing to provide heroic measures is reflected in "do not resuscitate" orders for elderly patients who do not wish to be revived in case of cardiac or respiratory arrest.

Failure to provide care to incompetent patients or to those who do not wish to be resuscitated conjures up the thought that there is such a thing as a life not worth living.[1] The ethical principle being espoused is that to provide care in these situations would in effect harm the patient but that to not provide care means the patient will die. The idea that death is better than life conflicts with many people's moral principles; this conflict is at the heart of many of the deepest, most emotional issues of our day. To some degree, even parts of the abortion controversy fall under this heading, since some people argue that the life of an unwanted baby would be worse than not living at all.

Because of the conflicts and differences of opinion, the obligation of the health care professional to do no harm is becoming more and more complicated in today's world. Only through a proper understanding of the patient's wishes (as defined through respect for autonomy) and through evaluation of what is in the patient's best interests (nonmaleficence versus beneficence) can ethical decisions be reached.[1]

Beneficence

While the lessons learned by studying nonmaleficence are important, the obligations of a health care professional go far beyond this concept. No one would ever seek medical care if the only promise were that no harm would be done. The APhA Code of Ethics exemplifies practice beyond nonmaleficence in that it requires pharmacists to render unto patients "the full measure of professional ability."

This is the concept of beneficence—to do good, to remove harms, to promote welfare. A corollary to the principle is that benefits and risks of therapy must be balanced. How are these concepts applied in pharmacy today?

Members of society are generally expected to render aid to those in need, but the obligations of a health care professional become larger because of the specialized knowledge possessed and because of the authority that society has given the professional. The health care professional is expected to render aid even when some degree of personal risk is involved. Just as a lifeguard is expected to rescue drowning swimmers at personal risk, the physician is expected to provide care to patients with infectious diseases, such as AIDS or hepatitis, at personal risk of acquiring those diseases.[1]

However, the professional's covenant cannot be activated unless both parties agree to its terms, and health care professionals do have some legal and ethical rights to select whom they will serve. Just because a patient has a need does not mean that the provider must care for that patient in nonemergency situations. Of course, legal restrictions would prevent physicians from discriminating on the basis of race, creed, color, nationality, or handicap. Diseases, including AIDS, have often been recognized as "handicaps," thus preventing health care professionals from refusing to care for patients with certain conditions.

The application of the principle of beneficence in health care often leads to conflict with respect to patient autonomy. The practice of paternalism in health care was the result of the provider unilaterally deciding what was in the best interest of the patient. This practice has now largely been replaced by the concept of respect for autonomy—that an informed patient is best able to choose from several potential therapies.

But this does not mean that the conflict between autonomy and beneficence has ended. Paternalism conflicts with respect for autonomy when a mentally unstable patient is not told that he or she has a terminal disease; here the patient is never given the information necessary to make an informed decision because the provider (the "father") believes that the patient would be incapable of rational thought or of making the best decision. Debate continues about how far health care professionals should be allowed to go in applying the principle of beneficence when it is in conflict with the patient's expressed or potential wishes.

The other key component of beneficence is the development of risk-benefit models that can be used to help with ethical decisions. In recent years, cost has been added to this model as the price of health care, especially medications, has risen dramatically in comparison with the costs of other goods in American society.

The evaluation of relative costs, benefits, and risks is based on the ethical theory of utilitarianism. It states that, given a choice between equally effective therapies, health care providers should seek to maximize benefits and minimize costs and risks. To analyze these three variables, various formal models of cost-effectiveness and cost-benefit analysis have been developed. Risk assessment is another technique used to focus on the amount of risk a patient would encounter in a given procedure.[1]

As students of algebra will recall, one cannot solve a single equation with two variables. Either one variable must be held constant or more information (another equation, in the algebraic problems) must be available. A similar line of thinking involves the ethical dilemmas of modern medicine: How can one select ethically from among different therapies that are equally effective but with different costs and risks? Or what processes can be used to choose between alternatives that are equally safe but with different costs and efficacies? In the final analysis, who will live and who will die? If the decision turns on costs and the relative wealth of the individual, has justice been done? That is the next element in ethical reasoning.

Justice

On first blush, the application of the principle of justice to health care makes one think of equal opportunity to obtain treatment for all people, regardless of wealth or social status. Despite its ethical appeal, this is probably not a realistic position, as some 40 million Americans have no health insurance, those with insurance must meet all kinds of conditions and copayments that they may not be able to afford, and only America's super-wealthy citizens could afford to pay their own health care bills throughout a lifetime.

So what is justice when it comes to health care? Aristotle noted that justice is the equal treatment of equals and the unequal treatment of unequals. But America purports to be a society of equals. Several major theories of justice are debated in America today:[1]

Table 5.2 | Six Stages of Moral Reasoning about Unauthorized Refills in Pharmacy Practice[a]

Classes of Morality	Stage No.	Example of Stage
Preconventional	1	Obedience: A pharmacist dispensing an unauthorized refill to avoid reprimands by owners of a pharmacy.
	2	Instrumental egoism and simple exchange: A pharmacist dispensing an unauthorized refill to do what he was being paid for and to give the patient what he wanted.
Conventional	3	Interpersonal concordance: A pharmacist dispensing an unauthorized refill because of a belief that the physician would be happy, the patient would be happy, and the pharmacy owner would be happy.
	4	Law and duty to the social order: A pharmacist dispensing an unauthorized refill only after calling the physician, or not dispensing it, because to do otherwise would be illegal.
Postconventional	5	Societal consensus: A pharmacist working with the pharmacy owner or nearby physicians to set up a system for handling unauthorized refills.
	6	Nonarbitrary social cooperation: Presented with a request for an unauthorized refill, a pharmacist dispensing it or refusing to dispense it based on the ultimate welfare of the patient.

[a] Adapted from reference 3.

- *Utilitarian theories of justice.* Justice is merely a form of the most paramount and stringent form of utility, so the system for evaluating risks, benefits, and costs must balance the private and public benefits, risks, and costs.
- *Libertarian theories of justice.* Individual liberty is the most important factor in libertarian thinking, so a free-market basis for health care is considered the most just. Perhaps even if people elect to buy and sell babies or organs for transplant, the libertarian would be happy so long as the government does not interfere with this expression of individual freedom.
- *Egalitarian theories of justice.* While not every person is entitled to an equal share of available goods and services, egalitarians believe that certain distributions of burdens and benefits should be equally available. This line of thinking serves to create basic rights for all citizens, some of which are stated (the right to vote) and some of which are implied (health care).

As the United States struggles to fix its ailing and very expensive health care system, the central problems will lie in the application of the principle of justice and the irreconcilable differences contained in the above three theories. So long as the financial resources of all citizens are not equal, it is certain that wealthier people will be able to seek medical interventions not available to other citizens. Perhaps a basic right to a certain minimum level of health care services will be identified, or perhaps a system of resource allocation or rationing on some other basis will be devised. Whatever the final decision, the application of the principle of justice along with respect for autonomy, nonmaleficence, and beneficence will keep medical ethicists busy for many years.

Ethical considerations in pharmacy practice

How do all these ethical principles translate into actual pharmacy practice? Like many theories, the information is more easily stated than applied. While the scope of this text does not allow detailed discussions of ethical dilemmas in pharmacy, many excellent analyses have been published in the medical and pharmacy literature. The *American Journal of Health-System Pharmacy* and *U.S. Pharmacist* have published much material on ethics in pharmacy over the years. Interested readers and classes should consult these for group discussions.

One article can assist in analyzing and categorizing pharmacy-related ethical principles. Dolinsky and Gottlieb[3] applied the model shown in Table 5.2 to pharmacy situations. The authors attribute actions taken in stages 1–3 as being primarily from self-interest, whereas stage 4 is legalistic. Stages 5 and 6 are based on principles and are more likely to be ethically proper—even though they may be illegal. As a practice exercise, describe ethical dilemmas that you have encountered while working in or visiting a pharmacy, and try to describe the stages of moral reasoning and the principles of ethics involved in the decision the pharmacist made.

Balancing the demands of society

As health care professionals with responsibility for the proper use of drugs in society, pharmacists are faced daily with ethical quandaries. Some of these are addressed in a minute-by-minute fashion, as patients and prescriptions come and go. Others develop over time, such as the physician who prescribes increasing amounts of narcotics for members of his or her family. Still others occur for pharmacists when they are fulfilling their roles as responsible members of a health care team or of the community (for example, offering advice to local governments about controlling illegal drugs). Without a moral and ethical framework within which to focus rational thought, pharmacists are at a loss in fulfilling their professional covenant with patients.

For pharmacy-specific examples of ethical situations, a good resource is APhA's textbook *Pharmacy Ethics: A Foundation for Professional Practice*.[4] It is available in print and online at www.pharmacylibrary.com.

REFERENCES

1. Beauchamp TL, Childress JF. *Principles of Biomedical Ethics*. 5th ed. New York, N.Y.: Oxford University Press; 2001.
2. Veatch RM. Hospital pharmacy: what is ethical? *Am J Hosp Pharm.* 1989;46(1):109–15.
3. Dolinsky D, Gottlieb J. Moral dilemmas in pharmacy practice. *Am J Pharm Educ.* 1986;50:56–9.
4. Buerki RA, Vottero LD. *Pharmacy Ethics: A Foundation for Professional Practice*. Washington, D.C.: American Pharmacists Association; 2013.

Chapter 6

Career Planning: Contemporary Pharmacy Practice Areas

Abir A. (Abby) Kahaleh

One of the great benefits of having a degree in pharmacy is the wide variety of career options that it opens to the individual. From going back to the corner drugstore in one's hometown to rising through the ranks of multinational corporate conglomerates, the possibilities are endless for the new pharmacy graduate.

In this chapter, the major areas of practice in pharmacy are presented along with strategies for career planning. In many pharmacy orientation courses, these brief oversights of practice areas are supplemented with presentations by guest lecturers who work in various practice settings. But don't let your investigation stop there—if an area of practice appeals to you, contact alumni from your school, faculty, preceptors, or local practitioners who work in that practice setting. If you decide on a path for your career, begin planning now so that you can take the elective courses that will give you a jump start after you graduate.

Before graduation, student pharmacists may face significant changes in the practice of pharmacy as the profession continues to evolve. Several recent studies have illustrated the benefits of pharmacist-provided services. Specifically, pharmacist-provided medication therapy management (MTM) enhanced medication adherence and reduced the costs of health care services. In 2014, a study by the Medicare Payment Advisory Commission showed that the adherent patient populations have significantly lower health care costs compared with the nonadherent populations.[1] Similarly, a 2013 report prepared for the Centers for Medicare & Medicaid Services concluded that patients with congestive heart failure, chronic obstructive pulmonary disease, and diabetes had consistently higher medication adherence rates after enrollment in Medicare Part D MTM programs.[2] Likewise, a 2013 study conducted by Avalere revealed that patients with higher adherence rate had lower mortality, reduced health care costs, and better health outcomes.[3] Finally, a 2012 research study that was published in *Health Affairs* indicated that a pharmacy-based intervention program increased the medication adherence rate among patients who received face-to-face counseling from pharmacists compared with those who received their medications and counseling by telephone from mail-service pharmacies.[4]

Although pharmacists are qualified to provide high-quality patient care services that reduce overall health care costs, they are not recognized as health care providers by third-party payers, including Medicare and Medicaid. Practitioners, faculty, and student pharmacists in the American Pharmacists Association (APhA) and other organizations have been leading the provider status initiative. Currently, pharmacists and pharmacists' patient care services are not included in the Social Security Act under Medicare Part B. Therefore, the lack of recognizing pharmacists as providers limits Medicare beneficiaries' access to pharmacist-provided services in ambulatory care settings. Consequently, health plans indicate that because of the lack of access to pharmacists' patient care, many beneficiaries do not receive needed comprehensive services during the transition from one care setting to another in integrated health care systems.[5]

Learning Objectives

Upon completion of this chapter, the reader should be able to:

1. Compare and contrast career options in pharmacy.

2. Examine critical factors that influence the selection of a pharmacy pathway.

3. Identify strategies for gaining knowledge about various pharmacy practice settings.

4. Describe advantages and disadvantages for each career option.

"In youth my wings were strong and tireless,
But I did not know the mountains.
In age I knew the mountains
But my weary wings could not follow my vision—
Genius is wisdom and youth."

—Epitaph of Alexander Throckmorton, from *Spoon River Anthology,* by Edgar Lee Masters

In addition to APhA efforts to expand access to pharmacists' patient care services under Medicare, other strategies have been used to increase pharmacists' services for Medicaid beneficiaries, such as changing the Medicaid programs in the Health Insurance Exchanges formed under the Affordable Care Act. Specifically, advocacy efforts have been made to expand access to pharmacist patient care services in accountable care organizations, patient-centered medical homes, commercial health plans, private insurance, and self-insured employers.[1]

In summary, APhA's efforts aim to assure that:

- Payers and policy makers recognize pharmacists as health care providers who improve access, quality, and value of health care.
- Access and coverage for pharmacists' patient care services are facilitated through Medicare and Medicaid, other federal and state health benefit programs, integrated care delivery models, and private payers.
- Pharmacists are included as members of health care teams.

One caveat is in order at this point in pharmacy history: Times are changing. As you learned in Chapter 3, MTM and pharmacists' patient care services are becoming more common in various pharmacy practices, and no one knows now what practice will be like in a few years. Likewise, the availability of increasingly sophisticated robotic equipment, informatics, and computerized systems along with the growing number of certified pharmacy technicians are affecting the practice of pharmacy in all settings. If pharmacists succeed in their advocacy initiatives, being recognized as providers could be a key factor that changes pharmacy practice by the time this edition of this textbook goes out of print. At a minimum, pharmacists' daily activities should be greatly different in a few years, and I discuss this possibility at appropriate places in this chapter.

Identifying a career option in pharmacy

A successful career is built on two things: good planning and good luck. And one of my favorite quotes is "The harder I work, the luckier I get."[6]

Although one never knows precisely when certain unique opportunities may be available, the wide variety of pharmacy positions available in many different settings can accommodate many plans for advancement throughout a career. And without planning, one will not be ready to seize the opportunities when they do arise.

Although every aspect in career planning could not be presented in any one book, the best advice to the student pharmacist is to find a good mentor. Identify the pharmacy faculty members in your school who seem knowledgeable about the parts of pharmacy that interest you, and ask them to give you advice on what courses and experiences will best prepare you for that career. Ask about personality inventory tests or other assessment tools that may be available for identifying your strengths and interests. Find out whether advanced study beyond your entry-level degree will be needed, and ask yourself whether you are willing or able to devote the extra time, investment, and energy for more studies. Learn whether you would be required to relocate for that career, and talk with your spouse, significant other, or family about what that might mean. With proper advice, input, and thought, your career choices should become obvious.

An important tool available to student pharmacists for career planning is the Pathways Evaluation Program for Pharmacy Professionals. Originally developed by Glaxo (now GlaxoSmithKline) in the 1980s, this program was transferred to APhA in 2001. An APhA Pathways Evaluation Program for Pharmacy Professionals Workshop Workbook and an assessment tool are available online.[7] It helps student pharmacists as well as pharmacists considering a career switch evaluate the importance to the individual of several critical factors that vary among pharmacy practice settings (Figure 6.1):[8]

- Interaction with patients
- Conducting physical assessments
- Interpreting laboratory values
- Continuity of relationships
- Helping people
- Collaboration with other professionals
- Educating other professionals
- Variety of daily activities
- Multiple task handling
- Problem solving
- Focus on expertise
- Innovative thinking
- Applying scientific knowledge
- Applying medical knowledge
- Creating new knowledge by conducting research
- Management/supervision of others
- Management/supervision of a business
- Pressure/stress
- Work schedule
- Part-time opportunities
- Job-sharing opportunities
- Exit/reentry opportunities
- Parental leave opportunities
- Leisure/family time
- Job security
- Opportunities for advancement
- Opportunities for leadership development
- Community prestige
- Professional involvement
- Income
- Benefits (vacation, health, retirement)
- Geographic location
- Autonomy
- Self-worth
- Future focus
- Professional prestige
- Unique practice environment
- Advanced degree
- Entrepreneurial opportunity
- Additional training
- Interaction with colleagues

Figure 6.1 | Critical job factors for pharmacy careers. Use this chart to ask yourself what you feel is important in your future pharmacy career.

Glaxo Pathway Evaluation Program for Pharmacy Professionals *Self-assessment Decision-Making Chart*		
Critical Job Factors	**Present Position**	**Optimal Position**
Counseling Spend time with patients, public		
Continuity of Relationships Maintain ongoing, long-term patient, consumer contact		
Helping People Directly or indirectly add to well-being of individuals, society		
Professional Interaction Involvement with other health care professionals		
Educating Other Professionals Time devoted to educating other health care professionals		
Repetition Very repetitive daily activities, tasks		
Multiple Task Handling Juggle many tasks at a time with interruptions		
Problem-solving Solve problems with tried, true solutions; or by exploring untested solutions		
Focus of Expertise Specialist or generalist		
Innovative Thinking Generate new ideas about pharmacy, pharmaceuticals		
Applying Scientific Knowledge Applying scientific or medical knowledge		
Business Management Organize, manage, assume risks of business		
Pressure Deal with crisis, quickly interpret medical, technical information		
Work Schedule Regular vs. irregular, long hours		
Leisure/Family Time Little vs. ample time for family, leisure activities		
Job Security Secure position and income		
Opportunity for Advancement Limited vs. many advancement opportunities		
Community Prestige Opportunity to gain recognition in the community		
Professional Prestige Opportunity to gain recognition in the profession		
Income Income level to meet lifestyle expectations		

Source: Adapted with permission from Sogol EM. *Career planning: gateway to future success.* US Pharm. 1990;(Oct):98–103.

- Travel
- Writing
- Working with teams
- Being "on call"
- Working on holidays
- Working on weekends
- Presentations

Additional materials can be accessed in the Careers Center on the APhA website (www.pharmacist.com/career-center). The online version of the Pathways evaluation allows you to rate 48 different factors that are similar to those shown in Figure 6.1 on a 1–10 scale. Based on these responses, the specific positions and work settings most likely to fit your responses are identified, along with detailed information about each.

Descriptions of various pharmacy practice settings are also available in the Student Center of the website of the American Association of Colleges of Pharmacy (www.aacp. org/resources/student/Pages/default.aspx).

Getting ready to pursue a career

One of the best ways to determine if you like a certain part of pharmacy is to work in that setting. Luckily, many possible options are available for doing that if you will look around and be willing to go where the job is.

Gaining this work experience is important in three ways: it provides you with the chance to see what your daily activities would be like in that setting, your experience there makes your school work more relevant by showing you why you need to know "all this stuff", and your commitment to that career option will appear stronger to potential employers when you are graduating. You should also remember that the time you spend searching for a job after you graduate is money lost—and your postgraduate salary will be many times greater than what you can make during school! Taking a lower-paying job during school to aid your career planning could be an important investment in your future.

If you are considering a career in pharmacy practice in community, hospital, or consultant pharmacy, positions should be available in your area. Talking with faculty members who deal a lot with alumni, looking in the newspaper, or visiting local pharmacies (or hospital pharmacies) can all be productive. To identify consultant pharmacists, you may need to contact the American Society of Consultant Pharmacists (ASCP) at the address shown in Table 6.1 and Chapter 8, because these are often **closed-shop pharmacies** located in industrial parks or office complexes.

For jobs in alternative pharmacy career paths, investigate the possibility of summer internships (Table 6.1). For instance, the APhA–ASP sponsors a summer internship program in the pharmaceutical industry. Student pharmacists from all over the United States work at various major research-oriented pharmaceutical companies for the summer. There, the students rotate through all the major parts of the company, learning about research and development of new drugs, marketing, sales, drug information, and professional relations.

Closed-shop pharmacies:
A pharmacy not open to the public. It usually provides services to nursing homes or other types of long-term care facilities. These services may be drug dispensing, consulting on patients' drug therapy, or both.

Table 6.1 | Contact Persons for Internship Programs

Industry	Contact
Pharmaceutical industry	Contact your dean or the advisor of your Academy of Students of Pharmacy Chapter for an application. Deadline for applications: November 30 of each year
Federal pharmacy	*COSTEP* Public Health Service Recruitment www.fda.gov Deadline for summer applications: December 31 of each year
Drug information	*United States Pharmacopeial Convention* www.usp.org Deadline for summer applications: February 1 of each year *National Council on Patient Information and Education* www.talkaboutrx.org Deadline for summer applications: March 1 of each year
Association management	*American Pharmacists Association* www.pharmacist.com Deadline for summer application: February 1 of each year *National Community Pharmacists Association* www.ncpanet.org Deadline for summer applications: April 15 of each year *American Society of Health-System Pharmacists* www.ashp.org Deadline for summer applications: February 1 of each year *Paul G. Cano Legislative Internship, American Society of Consultant Pharmacists* www.ascp.com (call to determine availability and schedule)
Pharmacy fraternities	*Phi Delta Chi* (www.phideltachi.org) and *Lambda Kappa Sigma* (www.lks.org) have periodically offered summer internships.

Likewise, the Public Health Service has COSTEP (Commissioned Officer Student Training and Extern Program). This three-month experience is available for student pharmacists to learn more about the role pharmacists can play in the federal government, including the Food and Drug Administration, the Indian Health Service, the Public Health Service, and the National Institutes of Health.

For student pharmacists who are intrigued by a career working in pharmacy associations, summer internships are available from APhA, the National Community Pharmacists Association (NCPA), the American Society of Health-System Pharmacists (ASHP), and periodically the pharmacy fraternities Lambda Kappa Sigma and Phi Delta Chi. All these are approximately three-month stints at the headquarters of these groups that involve rotations in various aspects of association work: membership, financial, conference planning, legal, executive support, editorial, and marketing. The NCPA and ASHP rotations are open to all student pharmacists; the fraternity groups generally choose from among their own members.

Experiences focused more on the provision of drug information as a career are available at the United States Pharmacopeial Convention and the National Council on Patient Information and Education.

In addition to the nationally oriented experiences shown in Table 6.1, many state pharmaceutical associations have part-time, temporary, and summer positions available. Ask your pharmacy school faculty about those possibilities.

These experiences can be critical in knowing beforehand whether certain areas of pharmacy are for you. Valuable postgraduate time can be saved by experiencing a part of pharmacy before entering the workplace, even if you learn that your expectations were not met and that another segment of the profession is more appealing.

One final point about career planning. Figure 6.2 shows the kinds of skills that will be needed in various parts of a pharmacy career, pretty much regardless of where you practice. Pharmacy school is designed to teach you much of the technical aspects of the profession; it touches only slightly on people and big-picture skills. Throughout your career, people skills will be very important; you must learn how to live, work, and communicate with others. As you are promoted throughout your career, what you learned in school will become less important than keeping the big picture in mind. This all means that you can never stop learning and that you should take advantage now of opportunities to advance your people skills. The best place to do that in pharmacy school is through involvement in student organizations, where you can learn about small-group decision making, conflict resolution, communication, teamwork, and goal setting.

With that background, let's look at the major areas of practice within pharmacy:
- Independent community pharmacy
- Chain pharmacy
- Institutional pharmacy
- Consultant pharmacy
- Managed, specialty, or home care
- Pharmaceutical industry, government, and associations

Figure 6.2 | **Pharmacy, people, and big picture skills needed in various levels of pharmacy management.**

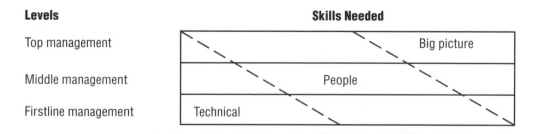

Source: Adapted with permission from Lorber RL, Weltner JC. *Productivity: balancing technical, people, and big picture skills.* Consult Pharm. 1987;2:196–8.

For each of the preceding areas of pharmacy practice, the following components will be addressed during each synopsis:

- Definition and scope of practice
- Position availability
- Salary
- Typical day
- Common rewards and frustrations
- Prospects of growth and advancement

Independent community pharmacy

As related in Chapter 2 on the history of pharmacy, the independent pharmacy is where the profession began, and it is still in many ways the heart and soul of pharmacy. Many of today's pharmacists came into the profession because of the respect they had for "doc" at the corner drugstore; in fact, for a sizable fraction of pharmacists, "doc" was their father or some other close relative. The spirit of entrepreneurship and the American dream of owning one's own business lives on in our country's 25,000 independent pharmacies, which have endured through decades of increasing competition from larger, better financed chain stores and decreasing reimbursement levels that have led to lower profit margins.

For independent pharmacists, the key word is *independent*. Pharmacists who choose to practice in independent community pharmacy are uniquely able to practice their profession in the way they choose, and this means they can more quickly transition their practices into MTM and pharmacists' patient care services if they choose to do so. They are able to respond quickly to changing consumer needs and have a real and lasting impact in their community. Through independent pharmacy, each practitioner has the opportunity to succeed or to fail. Each practitioner has the privilege—and the risk that comes with it—of setting the rules and determining the policies for the pharmacy.

According to the *NCPA Digest*, sponsored by Cardinal Health, independent community pharmacies include all pharmacist-owned and privately held businesses.[9] Independent pharmacies comprise single-store and pharmacist-owned pharmacies, including chain, franchise, compounding, long-term care, specialty, and supermarket units.[4] In 2012, about 14% of pharmacies had a total sales of $6.5 million, 29% reported sales in the range of $3.5 million to $6.5 million. Twenty percent of participating pharmacies indicated that their total sales were between $2.5 million and $3.5 million, and 37% reported sales under $2.5 million.[4]

In 2012, the independent community pharmacy accounted for $88.7 billion of the marketplace.[4] Most (91%) sales were from prescription medications. Despite the decreasing profit margins and payments from third-party payers, independent community pharmacists continue to use efficient business practices and provide valuable services to empower pharmacists and patients.[10]

Pharmacist positions are available in independent stores, and the country is filled with success stories for those who want to compete in this environment. Profiles of successful community pharmacists are published regularly in the NCPA magazine, *America's Pharmacist* (www.americaspharmacist.net; membership required), and APhA's *Phar-*

macy Today (www.pharmacytoday.org; open access) profiles a successful patient care services practitioner—including many in independent pharmacy practice—in each issue. Although starting salaries in independent pharmacies are often a little lower than in chain pharmacies, the prospects for advancement are different, especially if there is a chance to buy the pharmacy or start one's own pharmacy at some point.

All industries tend to go through three stages of development: sales growth, multiple locations, and diversification. Independent community pharmacy is no different. Most successful community pharmacies today have either several locations, which increases the company's sales and buying power, or diverse services, such as compounding, veterinary pharmacy, home care, **durable medical equipment**, long-term care (nursing homes or residential care facilities), or intravenous therapy. The growth possibilities in these emerging areas of patient care services and health care are limitless.

For pharmacists in entry-level positions in independent community pharmacy, much of the day is spent in drug-dispensing and patient-counseling activities. Many community pharmacies have pharmacy technicians who assist the pharmacist with the filling of prescriptions for checking and dispensing by the pharmacist. Computers are tremendously important in today's community pharmacy, because they have enabled pharmacies to provide advanced services, such as keeping **patient profiles**, checking for drug interactions, and providing patient-specific information for counseling, billing, drug-use review, or insurance purposes. Patient care services are facilitated in some computer software packages, including conducting and documenting medication therapy reviews, providing patients with a personal medication record, and generating medication-related action plans that are shared with physicians and other primary care providers.[11] The community pharmacist may compound special prescriptions for patients or prepare drugs for intravenous administration. As pharmaceutical care, MTM, and patient care services have become the norm and patient counseling is provided more universally in pharmacy, the pharmacist is spending increasing fractions of his or her time in direct patient care. This trend is making the pharmacist a source of primary care, thus making communication skills, patient-assessment techniques, and clinical knowledge all the more important.[12-15]

For managers or owners of community pharmacies, time is spent ordering merchandise and drugs, dealing with cash flow and accounts receivable or payable, handling personnel problems, marketing clinical and consulting services offered by the pharmacy, and planning for the future. Of course, since most independent pharmacies are small businesses, any employee may be called on to do almost anything—from managing the store while the owner is out of town to mopping the floors.

Practice in independent community pharmacies can be very rewarding for pharmacists who like to really know their patients, are attracted by the excitement of entrepreneurship that small businesses provide, or want the flexibility of finding a job in their hometown or virtually any other city or hamlet in the country. Independent pharmacists deal directly with the public, and they sometimes complain about some of those interactions, especially patients' criticisms about the skyrocketing prices of prescription drugs and problems with third-party payers. The pharmacist here feels caught in the middle, since the prices are dictated by the pharmaceutical manufacturer and the policies set by insurance companies and pharmacy benefits managers. The situation has been

Durable medical equipment: Items such as wheelchairs, walkers, and bedside toilets that patients buy when their health fails or rent during rehabilitative periods after surgery or injury. The term can also include various types of intravenous (also called parenteral) or enteral services that require special catheters or pumps to deliver fluids or nutrition through the patient's veins or the gastrointestinal tract safely.

Patient profiles: A record, usually computerized, of all medications a patient has received at a given pharmacy. Ideally, the profiles should include both prescription and nonprescription medicines.

compounded further by pharmaceutical companies that have become "whipping boys" in the public discourse for their pricing and marketing practices. Combined with the long hours of standing on one's feet with few breaks to even go to the restroom—much less sit down to eat—some pharmacists have experienced frustration in community independent pharmacy.

The entrepreneurial spirit definitely lives on for the pharmacy owner. In addition to a salary, the owner may benefit financially from the profits of the business, and he or she can sell the store when the time comes to retire or move on to some other situation.

All in all, independent community pharmacy provides a nice home for thousands of American pharmacists. Because of the nature of owning one's own business, many of these pharmacists are leaders in the profession, and they face today's challenges with just as much resolve, grit, and determination as did their predecessors who fought back intrusions by the merchants and grocers in Renaissance England.

Chain community pharmacy

Chain community pharmacists practice in cities and towns of all sizes and shapes and in a variety of settings, including the traditional chain pharmacy (such as CVS, Walgreens, and Rite Aid), supermarkets, and mass merchants (such as Target and Walmart). Chain pharmacies often have a large selection of merchandise in the front of the store; the pharmacy is often placed in back of the store to encourage consumers to pick up other items while they are getting their prescriptions filled.

Although the day-to-day operations of a prescription department are similar to those in independent pharmacies, a chain pharmacist is part of a larger corporate structure that provides numerous personal growth and career-development opportunities.[16]

A total of 115 corporate chains are members of the National Association of Chain Drug Stores (NACDS). According to the NACDS, chains operate more than 48,000 pharmacies (Table 6.2).[17] The chains include regional companies, which have at least four stores, and national operations. The chains employ 3.2 million persons, including 179,000 pharmacists. A total of 2.9 billion prescriptions are dispensed every year in chain pharmacies.

Table 6.2 | NACDS Chain Member Pharmacies

	1990	1995	2006	2016
Traditional	16,970	17,004	19,535	29,435
Supermarket	1,336	3,148	9,552	11,164
Mass Market	2,451	4,286	7,144	8,138
Total	20,757	24,438	36,231	48,737

Source: National Association of Chain Drug Stores.

Even though the perception of a chain drug store typically is that of a large retail out-let carrying a wide variety of merchandise, about two of every three NACDS members are small chains, meaning they operate at least four but no more than 50 stores. Many of these small chains operate like a typical independent pharmacy by carrying limited merchandise and focusing almost entirely on providing health-related products and services.[16]

The NACDS website (www.nacds.org) contains basic information and contact information for its member companies. If you're looking for a job or a career in chain community practice, this is a great place to start. The largest members of NACDS include Walgreens, CVS, Walmart, Rite Aid, Good Neighbor, Health Mart, Target, Publix, K-Mart, and Medicine Shoppe International.[18]

More than half of new pharmacy graduates enter chain practice each year. Reasons for this high proportion include job availability in nearly any part of the country, excellent salary and fringe benefit packages, store locations in areas of high population density, and the opportunity to interact with the public in a health care environment. New chain pharmacies are opening every day as they battle for market share in a competitive field. Chain pharmacists can expect to dispense an average of about 180 prescriptions per day in the typical chain pharmacy, based on national data available on the NACDS website.[18]

The front-line or staff pharmacist practicing in a chain pharmacy, no matter what the size, is afforded one of the greatest opportunities for patient interaction, if they can extract themselves from the prescription-filling process and find time for patient counseling and MTM. High-prescription-volume pharmacies heavily use trained technicians and automation to provide pharmacists with the time to counsel patients on their drug therapy and answer their questions.

Chain community pharmacies have led the pharmacy profession in developing the computer technology needed to keep up with the growing number of medications being used by patients each year. Sophisticated software programs have been developed by chains to maintain each patient's complete medication profile record and detect any potential drug interactions that could occur when a new drug is added to that profile. Online verification of a patient's eligibility under a specific insurance plan results in significantly reduced paperwork and handling of claims. Inventory control and pricing accuracy also are greatly enhanced by this heavy reliance upon computers.

A primary key to a satisfying career as a chain pharmacist is the continual contact with patients. As one chain pharmacist stated, "I've found that the key to good pharmacist–patient rapport lies in never losing sight of the patient's needs and perspective. To make sure this happens, it's important to be sympathetic to their conditions. With many of my older customers, the communication between us is just as important as the medications they use."

Numerous chain pharmacists become active in local, state, and national pharmacy associations, and typically chain employers are highly supportive when their pharmacists have opportunities to serve in leadership positions in these organizations or on state boards of pharmacy. Countless chain pharmacists actively support the educational programs of nearby pharmacy schools by serving as preceptors of student externs. Some chain pharmacists even serve as practitioner members of various schools' curriculum committees.

Many chains are expanding their scope of services into other health-related areas such as MTM, immunizations, nutrition and weight-loss programs (including some in which supermarket pharmacists take patients on shopping tours of the grocery store and teach them how to read food labels and plan their diets), home health care, nursing-home consulting, and home infusion therapy. This further increases the professional opportunities that await pharmacists who choose to practice in a corporate chain setting. Most chains have established pilot programs in MTM, and some have had hundreds of their pharmacists become certified in MTM delivery and/or immunizations. If these initial efforts take hold and the payment for services becomes routine, the face of pharmacy practice will be changed in the coming years.

A growing area in most corporate chain pharmacy organizations is the managed care department. Here, pharmacists negotiate contracts with health maintenance organizations, employer groups, and pharmacy benefit managers. In a chain pharmacy's purchasing department, pharmacists work with vendors and with generic and research-based pharmaceutical manufacturers in making drug-product-selection decisions.

Some pharmacists become so interested and involved in corporate management that they leave the pharmacy and health service division of their company and are promoted into positions in general merchandising, store layout and design, and even site selection and real estate negotiations. For those pharmacists who want to combine their professional talents with the challenge of the fast-paced retail business, numerous middle- and upper-level management positions are available. Many chains offer management training programs and specialized educational support that can help pharmacists chart a path that leads from the prescription department to one of several career tracks in management at the store, district, regional, and corporate levels.

Terminal position:
A position in a corporate hierarchy from which one has little hope for advancement because of an individual's education and corporate policies.

Pharmacists in chain practice are satisfied by the level of job security, the provision of continuing education directly by the employer, and the predictability that a corporate environment gives their careers and their personal lives. Practice can be just as rewarding in terms of patient contact if the pharmacist is allowed to practice professionally based on corporate policies and workload. The frustrations of patients complaining about prescription prices is worse in chains, because the patients there are more often bargain shoppers who are looking to save money. At the local level, pharmacists are sometimes frustrated by nonpharmacist store managers, who may interfere with the pharmacist's professional obligations to the patient. And frustration can result from reaching a **terminal position** early in one's career but being frozen into that position by the high salaries offered by chains.

The largest group of pharmacy graduates, year in and year out, goes directly into chain community pharmacy. Many of these people find a satisfying career there that gives them a lifetime of professional growth and opportunity. As the role of pharmacists in public health continues to expand, more student pharmacists are completing the APhA Pharmacy-Based Immunization Delivery certification program in school, and chain pharmacists are developing "immunization neighborhoods."

In 2013, the APhA Chief Strategy Officer Mitchell C. Rothholz provided an update on pharmacy immunization activities to the CDC Advisory Committee on Immunization Practices. The presentation highlighted the immunization process of care, legal and regulatory considerations and barriers, scope of immunization activities, best practices, documentation and communication processes, and innovations in the horizon for pharmacists' immunization activities, according to information on the APhA website, www.pharmacist.com.

In 2016, the CDC collaborated with NACDS by providing an $800,000 grant to fund innovative health care initiatives that demonstrate increased rates of pharmacy-based immunizations, including influenza, pneumococcal, pertussis, and herpes zoster. The grant aims to improve pandemic planning among pharmacies and state health departments and to enhance access to human papillomavirus vaccine educational programs and resources for pharmacists. These and other developments are making the pharmacy—and especially the chain community pharmacy—an increasingly important part of the nation's vaccination infrastructure.

Institutional pharmacy

Institutional pharmacy, traditionally practiced in hospitals and other "organized" health care settings, offers a diverse realm of possibilities to the new pharmacy graduate. Within today's disparate corporate hospital-based structures, an entire spectrum of pharmacist positions can be found in institutional pharmacy. Dispensing-only jobs require little contact with patients or other professionals outside the pharmacy, other than via telephone. Clinical pharmacy (analogous to MTM in community pharmacies) was born in hospitals, and positions with full-time clinical responsibilities are available on patient care units where interactions with physicians, nurses, and the rest of the **health care team** go on continuously. And there is management, dealing with multimillion-dollar personnel and drug budgets that can make or break the sales goals of pharmaceutical industry representatives in the area. If that is not enough, separate divisions and corporations exist for home care, outpatient pharmacies, drug information, drug research, and nutritional therapy.

Health care team:
A group of professionals with various skills who work together in providing patient care.

A definition of hospital or institutional pharmacy is therefore difficult. The primary commonality is that all the segments are part of a corporate structure that has grown since the 1950s, when the federal government funded the Hill-Burton Act for building new hospitals, and since 1966, when Medicare and Medicaid reimbursement began under Lyndon Johnson's Great Society program.

Jobs in hospital pharmacy are easy to find, but one needs to consider carefully what terminal position is desired. In 1963, hospital pharmacy began accrediting residencies (see Chapters 7 and 10), and today many jobs—especially management positions in the pharmacy—require that applicants have completed such a residency. If one wants to leap from the pharmacy into hospital administration, an appropriate master's degree (e.g., in business or hospital administration) would likely be needed. Large hospitals are often affiliated with schools of medicine or pharmacy, and most clinical positions require a PharmD degree plus postgraduate residencies, fellowships, or both. One's career in hospital pharmacy, particularly in larger institutions, can thus be greatly affected by decisions made as a student or young practitioner.

Chapter 6

Salaries in hospital pharmacy have historically been somewhat lower than in community pharmacy, especially in chain pharmacies. That may be true to some degree still, but the gap has been largely closed as a result of pharmacist shortages in the late 1990s and early 2000s. The possibilities for advancement are strong in this field, and more than a few hospital pharmacy directors have been promoted into hospital executive positions. In these, they are administratively responsible for numerous departments that can range from the clinical laboratory to materials management or housekeeping. For an employee who is not at financial risk (as would be an independent pharmacy owner), the salaries of hospital pharmacy director and executive positions are high. However, because of the pyramidal shape of hospital pharmacy staffs, the competition for management positions can be keen.

Benefits in hospitals tend to be very favorable, compared with other parts of pharmacy. This resulted from the large number of employees in hospitals, including some unionized groups that have demanded and received favorable benefits packages over the years.

For the pharmacist whose responsibilities are centered on drug distribution, the daily mission is to get the right drugs to the right patient at the right time. Most hospitals employ pharmacy technicians who assist greatly with this task. These technicians are quite capable, many of them having weeks or months of training, years of experience, and certification from the Pharmacy Technician Certification Board. In some hospitals, technicians are responsible for providing the **controlled substances** to nursing units and for making intravenous solutions for patient administration.

Clinical pharmacists in the hospital are involved in more patient care and drug information activities. Some pharmacists **"round"** with the health care team, which comprises physicians, nurses, respiratory therapists, social workers, and physical or occupational therapists. Other pharmacists provide care to patients who need specialized pharmacy services, such as **pharmacokinetic monitoring** or **nutrition support**. Some larger institutions have drug information centers, where pharmacists answer questions from health care professionals or the public about drugs, poisonings, and medication use.

Institutional pharmacy administrators in midsize and larger facilities have a life similar to that of midlevel managers in many corporations. Little time is spent in direct pharmacy practice; life instead is personnel schedules and problems, budgeting, purchasing, and dealing with situations ranging from medication errors to pharmacists or technicians stealing controlled substances for personal use or street sale. As mentioned earlier, a fair number of pharmacist managers are able to rise into hospital administration after they have obtained master's degrees in either business administration or hospital administration.

Most pharmacists seem to either love or hate hospital practice. In pharmacy school, hospital pharmacy is sometimes glorified because of the important role it has played in creating the clinical pharmacy and pharmaceutical care movements, which led to the establishment of MTM in community pharmacies. But the hospital is threatening to some—it is a large building with hundreds or thousands of employees and patients. Introductory and advance pharmacy practice experiences may consist of helping pharmacy technicians fill **patient carts** with **unit dose packages** of drugs in a windowless basement pharmacy. The preceptor, often the director of pharmacy, may never be around, because he or she attends a seemingly endless string of committee meetings in other parts of the hospital. Thus, many student pharmacists or young pharmacists become turned off by hospital practice, based on a short but not necessarily representative experience.

But for those who love the institutional environment, the hospital is great. Many patients are quite ill, so the rewards are immediately apparent when the pharmacist attends a successful **code blue.** In larger hospitals, dozens of other pharmacists interact daily, and trading schedules or getting vacation time is easy. The hours are very predictable, usually one of three shifts: 7 am to 3 pm, 3 pm to 11 pm, or 11 pm to 7 am. However, many hospital pharmacies are open 24 hours a day each day of the year, and staffing requirements can lead to conflicts with pharmacists' personal lives.

The possibilities for professional growth in hospital pharmacy have been very good, and the largest pharmacy convention in the world is the American Society of Health-System Pharmacists' Midyear Clinical Meeting, which is held the first week of December each year. Up to 20,000 people regularly attend that meeting. With such a concentration of well-trained health care professionals, the hospital provides an intellectually stimulating atmosphere devoid of many of the frustrations one finds in community practice.

Disappointments in hospital pharmacy are similar to those alluded to above: feelings of isolation if confined to a basement pharmacy for drug distribution; difficulties with bureaucratic tendencies; and a lack of face-to-face patient contact for those without clinical responsibilities. Salaries are not overly aggressive because many people are willing to trade some of the advantages of hospital work for a slightly lower salary.

Institutional pharmacy practice continues to be a very exciting, dynamic area of practice. Virtually every kind of pharmacy practice can be found in hospitals somewhere: outpatient (ambulatory) pharmacy, acute care, emergency care, nuclear pharmacy (handling of radioactive drugs), long-term care, and home care. About 5,000–6,000 hospitals provide care in virtually all areas of the United States except the most rural or least populated. Hospital pharmacy has provided much of pharmacy's reprofessionalization over the past seven decades (see Chapter 3), and practice there can be very rewarding for those who prefer its environment.

Recently, several studies have revealed the expanding role of institutional pharmacists in the transition-of-care process. A study was conducted to examine the impact of expanding pharmacists' services in anticoagulation clinics.[19] The study concluded that pharmacist-provided counseling by telephone increased the number of visits to the clinic without adversely affecting patient outcomes or increasing health care costs. Another research study focused on examining a pharmacist-led antimicrobial stewardship program (ASP) without infectious disease physician support.[20] The results of the study indicated that ASP resulted in improved and efficient antimicrobial use. Another study focused on the implementation of clinical pharmacy services among pediatric patients on dialysis.[21] The results of the study showed that pharmacists improved the satisfaction and biochemical outcomes among patients.

Pharmacists have also been contributing to a new frontier, clinical pharmacy in emergency medicine.[22] Pharmacists are playing a key role in providing clinical services,

Patient carts:
Hospital pharmacies often use carts with small drawers, one for each patient on a nursing station, to deliver medications from a central or decentral pharmacy to the patient care floors. Each nursing-station cart is exchanged periodically, usually once a day, with a new supply of medications for each patient.

Unit dose packages:
In hospitals and some nursing homes, medications are packaged in strips, with each dose labeled with the brand name, strength, and generic name of the drug. Even though this packaging costs more, it speeds the pharmacy operation and permits return of unused medication to the pharmacy.

Code blue:
The hospital's response when a patient is in cardiopulmonary arrest (the heart and/or lungs have stopped). Various health care professionals respond to the code blue, and the pharmacist attends to help calculate doses and draw up drugs to be administered in this emergency situation. Hospitals differ in what they call the situation; code blue is a common term derived from the fact that the patient is turning blue from a lack of oxygen. Other names are code red or code 99.

including pharmacotherapy consults, drug information, toxicology recommendations, and microbiology culture reviews.

Long-term-care pharmacy

Another area of pharmacy practice with rich clinical opportunities is the provision of services to patients who are institutionalized in long-term-care facilities. Although nursing homes commonly provide this institutional care, a number of factors are leading to the establishment of many other kinds of facilities collectively known as community-based long-term care. In nursing homes, patients (or residents as they are called in this setting) are deficient in one or more of the normal activities of daily living: ambulating, eating, bathing and dressing, or toileting. In community-based long-term care, the resident may simply need assistance with taking his or her medications at the right time or with preparing meals. In fact, the resident may be living at home, and the long-term-care service may be a nurse or personal assistant who comes by once a day to help with such activities.

This is the world of the long-term-care pharmacist, who is also called a consultant pharmacist because the relationship between the facility or agency and the pharmacist is most often contractual (that is, the pharmacist consults to the facility under contract, rather than working as an employee of the nursing home). Consultant pharmacists work from a variety of settings, most of them remote from the nursing home or facility:

- Community independent or chain pharmacies that provide a limited amount of long-term care services
- Stand-alone long-term care pharmacies, owned either independently or by a chain pharmacy or large long-term care corporation
- Pharmacies that provide no drugs but only consult on the proper procedures and therapies in a facility
- Hospital pharmacies
- Pharmacies located in nursing homes (where the pharmacist may very well be an employee of the facility)

Consultant pharmacist services to nursing homes are mandated under federal law. To qualify for Medicaid reimbursement, a nursing home must have the drug regimens of all residents reviewed by a pharmacist each month. This clinical pharmacy service, first mandated in 1974, was the only one recognized in federal statutes until Congress began requiring pharmacists to counsel all Medicaid patients in 1990.

Salaries for consultant pharmacists usually start out between the independent/hospital range and the chain range. Some consultant pharmacists who own their own businesses have done extremely well; a survey of consultant pharmacists noted that one practitioner earned nearly $1 million annually. For pharmacists who work in consulting only, the salaries are good but do not start out as high as those in chain pharmacy. Consultant pharmacy has been a primary area of entrepreneurship in pharmacy since the late 1960s, and the employee who is willing to work harder can generally find an employer who is willing to pay for that dedication. However, the consultant pharmacy market consolidated during the 1990s, and entry-level pharmacists now often find themselves working for large corporations that are not unlike the large chain pharmacies in many ways.

There could very well be no such thing as a typical day for a consultant pharmacist, but there are typical months. Long-term care pharmacists who provide drug distribution have daily responsibilities very similar to those of hospital pharmacists. Working with technicians, the pharmacist responds to physician orders and other requests that come in from the nursing home; communication today is usually by fax or through computerized physician order entry systems. Drugs are provided to the facility, sometimes in specialized packaging that helps nurses organize their medications according to time of intended drug administration.

Some consultant pharmacists spend most or all of their time reviewing the drug regimens of residents. They often work for larger pharmacies that serve only nursing home and long-term-care facilities (closed-shop pharmacies, defined earlier in this chapter). Because these facilities may be located hundreds of miles apart, many consultant pharmacists spend a lot of time on the road, driving from one home to the next. This position can be very clinical, because all day long the pharmacist leaves notes for physicians requesting more laboratory testing, decreased medication doses, discontinuation of unnecessary or duplicative drugs, and addition of agents for previously unrecognized problems.

Other pharmacists rise into management or own consultant pharmacy operations. Their jobs are similar to managers in hospital or community pharmacy, with a very strong entrepreneurial spirit in this sector. In addition, the managers or owners are usually responsible for the never-ending process of marketing needed to maintain or expand one's business in this particular part of health care.

Many pharmacists have come to love consultant pharmacy. It combines the clinical aspects of hospital pharmacy with the patient contact and business challenges of community pharmacy. Conventions of the ASCP are simply exciting events, attended by people bubbling over to share their ideas and enthusiasm with colleagues facing similar situations. Even in the exhibits, attendees are not just looking to "fill up their bags with goodies"; instead, they genuinely seek information from exhibitors that will aid their practices. For many, consultant pharmacy is a dream come true.

Common frustrations with consultant pharmacy include the travel associated with monthly drug-regimen review and the lack of direct contact with the nurses and physicians caring for the residents. Because many residents of nursing homes are older or have incurable conditions (such as paraplegics or those with Alzheimer's disease), the work is not as dramatically rewarding as in the hospital. Nursing homes usually expect a pharmacist to be "on call" at night and on weekends, which could frustrate the pharmacist who values his or her personal time.

With Americans living longer and the huge baby-boom generation now reaching retirement age, consultant pharmacy will be a growing field in the coming decades. For the pharmacist looking for a career that fulfills the clinical promises of pharmacy, consultant pharmacy can be the answer.

Co-payment:
The amount of money a patient must pay when receiving certain types of health care services under insurance programs or prepaid health care plans.

Chronic conditions:
Diseases that last for more than about 6 months or that have long-term (usually lifelong) effects are referred to as chronic conditions. These include diabetes, hypertension (high blood pressure), and heart conditions. In addition, surgery and other therapies may produce a chronic condition. For instance, a colon cancer patient may have all or some of the colon removed, with an ostomy created for the passage of waste. Or a patient whose stomach is removed because of gastric cancer may require special types of enteral nutrition rather than a normal diet of solid foods.

Formulary:
A list of drugs that have been selected by the medical staff of a hospital or HMO for use in that institution. Drugs are selected on the basis of efficacy, safety, cost, and quality of life. In recent years, the marketing of many "me-too" drugs by the pharmaceutical industry—drugs that have no important advantage over drugs already on the market—has made cost an increasingly important factor in formulary decisions. Another important factor is the number of times per day that a medicine must be given, since in hospitals, highly paid personnel must dispense and administer each dose and in HMOs patient compliance is higher with fewer doses.

Managed care, home care, mail-service, and specialty pharmacy

Four other areas of pharmacist practice employ a small but increasing number of pharmacy graduates.

Managed care refers to health care provided by corporations such as health maintenance organizations (HMOs) or preferred provider organizations (PPOs). These corporations are really a form of insurance. They collect a prepaid premium from a consumer (or from the employer) and in return provide all needed health care services. Incentives are in place to shepherd patients to obtain the care from the organization's own employees (in the case of HMOs) or from designated physicians, hospitals, and other providers (in the case of PPOs). Access to certain kinds of care, especially psychiatric services or long-term care, may be limited. Other types of care, including pharmacy services, may require a **co-payment** by the patient at the time of service as a way of preventing overuse of the system.

Managed care grew rapidly during the 1990s as a way to contain health care costs. It is now an established practice setting. Some managed care companies are owned by the large pharmaceutical chains, and managed care provider organizations have their own in-house pharmacies that enrollees can use, usually with a lower or no co-payment.

PPOs contract with preferred community pharmacies to provide prescriptions on a fee or cost-plus-fee basis. Some PPOs offer incentives to patients who are on long-term drug therapy for **chronic conditions** such as hypertension to obtain such medicines from a mail-service pharmacy. These pharmacies, often located in other states, have been very controversial among pharmacists because they offer no opportunity for face-to-face patient–pharmacist contact and they take away the kinds of prescriptions that are the bread and butter for community pharmacies. However, with the advent of toll-free telephone numbers, e-mail communications, fax machines, computerized physician order entry systems, computerized patient-specific drug information, automated drug-dispensing technology, and overnight delivery services such as FedEx, the mail-service industry has been growing. For many elderly patients for whom travel is a major difficulty or an impossible chore, just the delivery of the medicine to the door is a critical plus—a fact that must be kept in mind by service-oriented pharmacists.

Some pharmacists work directly for managed care organizations, including the big insurers such as Aetna and United Health Group. They assist with **formulary** management, prior authorization of off-formulary and expensive medications, and other such tasks.

The home care market is centered on the specialized needs of patients who have a short- or long-term need for products such as intravenous antibiotic solutions, intravenous nutritional solutions, or enteral (via the mouth or stomach) nutritional feedings. Home health care services require the formation of a health care team, with nurses who visit patients in their homes periodically, respiratory therapists who set up home oxygen equipment or provide respiratory care services at home, pharmacists and pharmacy technicians who prepare solutions and monitor the patients' care, dietitians who consult on the patients' nutritional needs, and delivery personnel who transport all these goods to the patients' homes.

Because the managed and home care markets are growing rapidly and because students are not as familiar with these settings, pharmacist positions are plentiful. HMOs, which require a substantial population base, are common in all major cities of the United States. Home care can be found everywhere, and such services are especially critical in rural areas where patients may live without transportation in remote locations. The central pharmacy operation is sometimes in a major city, with delivery personnel who travel both in the city and to the rural areas, or the pharmacy may be located in small towns. Some community independent and chain pharmacies offer home care services from within a retail location.

Mail-service pharmacies are fewer in number and more geographically dispersed. They tend to be located near population centers. Some state boards of pharmacy have banned mail-service pharmacies, so those states do not have any pharmacies of this type.

Another type of pharmacy that generally relies on postal or overnight delivery services is the specialty pharmacy. As the pharmaceutical industry has developed increasingly sophisticated drug products—many of them from biological rather than chemical sources and intended to treat rare diseases—a need has arisen for limiting the number of pharmacies handling these specialized agents. Pharmacists working in specialty pharmacies know these drug well, understand how payment can be obtained for them, and are able to keep patients informed about when the medications will arrive at their homes and how the drugs must be stored and administered.

Salaries in managed care, home care, mail-service, and specialty pharmacies are very similar to other entry-level positions. Pay scales for entry-level chain pharmacy jobs are probably higher, but independent, hospital, and consultant positions would have salaries quite similar to those in this part of pharmacy.

For the managed care pharmacist, a typical day would be very similar to that in community pharmacy, but with key exceptions. Because the HMO pharmacist is located in a building with prescribers and institution-like policies and procedures are used, contact with the physician is both easy and productive. For instance, the HMO may have a formulary system, which is a medical staff policy that only certain drugs and drug products may be used for the HMO's patients. Thus, if a physician prescribes a nonformulary drug, the pharmacy may have been granted the authority by the medical staff to change that prescription to a safer, lower cost, or more effective drug that is on the formulary. Or, if the pharmacist wants to discuss the prescription with the prescriber, a face-to-face meeting may be only steps away.

Managed care pharmacists employed by the large payers often work virtually, usually from home offices. Working through dedicated websites or by e-mail, they spend much of their day responding to requests for approvals for medications, handling drug information questions, or preparing summaries of new drugs being considered for formularies.

Managers of HMO pharmacies face similar pressures as do hospital pharmacy administrators. All of these pharmacists operate within a hierarchical corporate structure that places a great deal of emphasis on costs and cost containment. Committee and department head meetings are common, and business skills are very advantageous for these administrative pharmacists.

In the home care arena, pharmacists' activities are similar to those in the intravenous product preparation area of a hospital pharmacy. If the pharmacy employs technicians, the pharmacist becomes more of a manager and clinical consultant on the care of the patients. Otherwise, the pharmacist would spend a fair amount of time in product preparation. Pharmacists in home care do travel periodically to provide pharmaceutical care to patients directly, but the distances involved limit this activity somewhat.

Staff-level positions in mail-service pharmacy are largely in quality control—making sure that the automated dispensing machines have correctly filled each prescription. The pharmacist sits at a work station next to a conveyor belt, and completed prescriptions in bins queue up there. After a scanner reads a bar code on the bin, the medication order—and many times a photograph of the prescribed tablet or capsule—appears on the pharmacist's computer screen. The pharmacist makes sure that the medication and the prescription label are correct and authorizes drugs to be mailed to the patient. Using such technology, a pharmacist can dispense several hundred prescriptions in an 8-hour shift.

Specialty pharmacists are also involved in delivering product, but they additionally have many patient education and payment responsibilities. This provides a nice mix of daily activities in this setting.

The opportunities for advancement in these areas are still being defined. Managed care, mail-service, and specialty pharmacy seem similar to the hospital environment because they provide job security but with somewhat limited potential for advancement. Home care is more entrepreneurial, making advancement to owning the business (or setting up a similar one) quite feasible. The pressures in each setting are just like those discussed earlier for hospital versus independent practice. The managed care pharmacist is usually part of a large department, with professional contact, schedule flexibility, and role specialization very common. The home care pharmacist is often in a smaller operation, meaning that he or she has a very diverse job. Finding someone to work on a given day may be difficult, particularly if the pharmacy is located in a rural area. But the home care pharmacy is not filled with the rules and regulations common to larger bureaucracies, such as the HMO.

For the pioneer pharmacist, managed care, home care, mail-service, and specialty pharmacy are currently the frontier of pharmacy practice. Depending on the direction health care takes, they could represent the future for an increasing number of pharmacists.

Other careers for pharmacists

Three other important career paths for pharmacists are in pharmaceutical industry, government, and associations. Although the skills and knowledge used in these jobs are only somewhat related to what students learn in pharmacy school, that background makes pharmacists ideal choices in many situations.

Pharmaceutical industry employs pharmacists in sales, marketing, government affairs, drug information, research, management, professional relations, and executive positions. Long-term (but maybe not starting) salaries and benefits can be higher in industry, and pharmacists who prefer a competitive, dynamic, and growing workplace like work with the industry. Many companies start pharmacists out "carrying the bag"—meaning as pharmaceutical representatives to physicians, hospitals, and pharmacies—but this is becoming less common. Promotions from sales positions are often into marketing or government affairs. Companies generally have a limited number of positions available in drug information, which is the part of the company that fields questions from health care professionals and the public.

For the student considering a career in pharmaceutical industry, the APhA–Academy of Student Pharmacists summer internship in industry is a must (see Table 6.1)—an absolute must! A commitment to a career in industry usually involves relocation, and reentry into more traditional types of pharmacy practice becomes impractical quickly. Thus, these summer internships are extremely valuable in assessing industry as a career option.

A variety of positions are possible for pharmacists in government. Federal organizations such as the U.S. Public Health Service, the Food and Drug Administration, and the Drug Enforcement Administration employ pharmacists, and several pharmacists work for senators and representatives in the U.S. Congress. Related agencies such as the Congressional Office of Technology Assessment sometimes need pharmacists for specific research projects that are assigned by Congress. In state governments, the agencies responsible for Medicaid and Medicare reimbursement and the State Board of Pharmacy employ pharmacists in management and enforcement positions. No one goes to work for the government because of the salaries, or even for the job stability these days. But the opportunity to influence public policy related to pharmaceuticals and pharmacy services is all that it takes for many pharmacists to become involved as public servants.

Pharmacists are also often elected to positions of leadership by their constituents. Pharmacists have served in the U.S. Senate and House of Representatives, and dozens are active in the statehouses. One pharmacist—Hubert H. Humphrey—even served as vice president and was the Democratic nominee for president in 1968. At the local level, pharmacists are often intimately involved with politics and other positions, including mayor, school board members, and city or county commissioners. As the best educated person in any community who is directly accessible to the public, pharmacists are very well-respected people.

The COSTEP program is a valuable opportunity for the student pharmacist who wants to see more about a career in government (see Table 6.1). It provides an introduction to the U.S. Public Health Service, which is a primary path for pharmacists who would like a career in government work (including the Indian Health Service, which has been very progressive in its pharmacy services). The Department of Veterans Affairs has implemented some exciting changes for both pharmacists employed at VA centers and those in distant communities.[16,18]

Another potential career path is in the field of association management. As is true for government, these positions are often located in Washington, D.C., or in the state capitals. In fact, most associations were started to influence the governmental oversight of a profession (see Chapters 7 and 8). Many very different kinds of positions make association work exciting: professional affairs (making policies about how pharmacists should practice or be educated); legal affairs (interfacing with the legislative, judicial, and executive branches of government to ensure the opportunity for pharmacists to provide quality pharmaceutical care); educational affairs (setting up conferences or study programs for pharmacists' continuing education); editorial work (writing or editing books, journals, software, and other pharmacy works); and executive activities (managing association offices and dealing with members who volunteer for leadership positions). Salaries in association work are not much higher than those in government, but the benefits are good, with travel to pharmacy conventions and lots of contact with colleagues a part of the job.

Although several internships are available in association management (see Table 6.1), students more often consider postgraduate, 12-month residencies in association management. These are available at ASHP, ASCP, and NCPA (see Chapter 8 for addresses and Chapter 10 for more information).

Many pharmacists find that their careers lead them into work with the industry, government, or associations. For these pharmacists, the rewards are very satisfying.

Pharmacy: A diverse profession

As described in this chapter, a degree in pharmacy opens the door to a dazzling array of career options. By studying the differences between various choices (Table 6.3), learning more about yourself (see Figure 6.1), and going out and meeting people working in the different parts of pharmacy practice, you can select the path that is just right for you.

Table 6.3 | Summary of Key Aspects of Pharmacy Practice Areas

| Practice Area | Key Satisfaction Factors[a] | | | |
	Job Availability	Salary	Advancement	Feeling of Accomplishment
Independent	S	S	S	+
Chain/grocery store/ mass merchandiser	+	+	S	−
Hospital	S	S	+	+
Consulting	S	S	+	+
Managed care	S	S	S	+
Home care	S	S	+	+
Mail service/specialty	−	S	S	−
Industry	S	+	S	S
Government	−	−	S	+
Associations	S	−	+	+

[a] Shown are the author's overall opinion of the relative level of satisfaction most pharmacists have with the factors shown in each area of pharmacy practice. Key to codes: + indicates greater than average level compared with other pharmacy jobs; S indicates an average level; − indicates below average level.

REFERENCES

1. Medicare Payment Advisory Commission. *Report to the Congress: Medicare Payment Policy.* Washington, D.C.: MedPAC; 2014. http://medpac.gov/documents/reports/mar14_entirereport.pdf. Accessed April 6, 2016.

2. *Medication Therapy Management in Chronologically Ill Populations: Final Report.* Burlingame, Calif.: Acumen LLC; 2013. https://innovation.cms.gov/files/reports/mtm_final_report.pdf. Accessed April 6, 2016.

3. Braithwaite S, Shirkorshidian I, Jones K, Johnsrud M. *The Role of Medication Adherence in the U.S. Healthcare System.* Washington, D.C.: Avalere Health; 2013. http://static.correofarmaceutico.com/docs/2013/06/24/adher.pdf. Accessed April 6, 2016.

4. Pringle JL, Boyer A, Conklin MH et al. The Pennsylvania Project: pharmacist intervention improved medication adherence and reduced health care costs. *Health Aff.* 2014;33(Aug):81444-52.

5. American Pharmacists Association. The pursuit of provider status: what pharmacists need to know. APhA Fact Sheet; September 13. www.pharmacist.com/sites/default/files/files/Provider%20Status%20FactSheet_Final.pdf. Accessed March 30, 2016.

6. Samuel Goldwyn Quotes. BrainyQuote.com website. www.brainyquote.com/quotes/quotes/s/samuel-gold122307.html. Accessed March 30, 2016.

7. APhA Pathways Evaluation Program for Pharmacy Professionals. APhA website. www.pharmacist.com/apha-career-pathway-evaluation-program-pharmacy-professionals. Accessed March 30, 2016.

8. Independent pharmacy today. National Community Pharmacists Association http://www.ncpanet.org. Accessed June 7, 2017.

9. National Community Pharmacists Association. *2013 NCPA Digest Financial: Community Pharmacy in the Digital Age.* Alexandria, Va.: NCPA; 2013. www.ncpanet.org/pdf/digest/2013/2013digest_financials.pdf. Accessed April 5, 2013.

10. Kahaleh AA, Gaither C. The effects of work setting on pharmacists' empowerment and organizational behaviors. *Res Social Adm Pharm.* 2007;3(2):199-222.

11. American Pharmacists Association and National Association of Chain Drug Stores Foundation. Medication therapy management in pharmacy practice: core elements of an MTM service model (version 2.0). *J Am Pharm Assoc.* 2008;48(3):341-53.

12. Fera T, Bluml BM, Ellis WM, et al. The Diabetes Ten City Challenge: interim clinical and humanistic outcomes of a multisite community pharmacy diabetes care program. *J Am Pharm Assoc.* 2008;48(2):181-90.

13. Bunting BA, Smith BH, Sutherland SE. The Asheville Project: clinical and economic outcomes of a community-based long-term medication therapy management program for hypertension and dyslipidemia. *J Am Pharm Assoc.* 2008;48(1):23-31.

14. Peacock G, Kidd R, Rahman A. Patient care services in independent community pharmacies: a descriptive report. *J Am Pharm Assoc.* 2007;47(6):762-7.

15. Nicholas A, Divine H, Nowak-Rapp M, Roberts KB. University and college of pharmacy collaboration to control health plan prescription drug costs. *J Am Pharm Assoc.* 2007;47(1):86-92.

16. National Association of Chain Drug Stores website. http://www.nacds.org. Accessed April 5, 2008.

17. Statement of the NACDS for U.S. House of Representatives Committee on Energy and Commerce Subcommittee on Health on "Examining the FY 2016 HHS Budget." http://www.nacds.org/pdfs/pr/2015/EC_HHS_Subcommittee_Budget_Testimony.pdf. Accessed April 6, 2016.

18. National Association of Chain Drug Stores website. http://www.nacds.org. Accessed April 5, 2008.

19. Philip A, Green M, Hoffman T, et al. Expansion of clinical pharmacy through increased use of outpatient pharmacists for anticoagulation services. *Am J Health Syst Pharm.* 2015;72(7):568-72.

20. Waters CD. Pharmacist-driven antimicrobial stewardship program in an institution without infectious disease physician support. *Am J Health Syst Pharm.* 2015;72(6): 466-8.

21. El Borolossy R, El Wakeel L, El Hakim I, Badary O. Implementation of clinical pharmacy services in a pediatric dialysis unit. *Pediatr Nephrol.* 2014;29(7):1259-64.

22. Acquisto NM, Hays DP. Emergency medicine pharmacy: still a new clinical frontier. *Am J Health Syst Pharm.* 2015;72(23);2092-6.

Chapter 7 | Governmental and Voluntary Oversight of Pharmacy

L. Michael Posey

Pharmacists are fond of saying that pharmacy is the most regulated profession in the United States, and, if it were possible to quantify this, the statement might indeed be true. Certainly no other traditionally mercantile-oriented occupation has the degree of controls on the selling of its goods as does pharmacy. But given the inherent danger of abuse of and addiction to many pharmaceutical products, society's interest in looking over pharmacy's shoulder is quite understandable and necessary. As pharmacy shifts from a product to a patient focus, pharmacists have actively and aggressively sought recognition by the federal government as a "provider", denoting a health care professional eligible to be paid for patient care services not associated with a product under health care programs of the federal government.

In addition to state and federal laws, pharmacy is increasingly responsive to oversight by a number of voluntary agencies and organizations. In institutions, pharmacy must meet certain standards to qualify for federal reimbursement for care delivered to Medicare and Medicaid patients. Colleges of pharmacy must meet certain criteria so that their graduates can be recognized as licensed pharmacists. Postgraduate residencies and fellowships follow standards set forth by various pharmacy associations or other accrediting agencies. And pharmacists working in specialized areas of the profession and pharmacy technicians can seek recognition for the special knowledge that they have gained.

How did this imposing structure of pharmacy regulation and oversight develop, and what does it mean today? Let's take a look.

Federal laws and regulations

A complex array of federal and state **laws** and **regulations** govern the practice of pharmacy. Some of the laws vary from state to state, and many state laws differ from federal pronouncements. A key rule to remember is that the more stringent law is the one that should be followed, regardless of its origin.

At the federal level, three agencies are of primary importance to pharmacy: the Food and Drug Administration (FDA), the Drug Enforcement Administration (DEA), and the Centers for Medicare & Medicaid Services (CMS, formerly the Health Care Financing Administration), which regulates payments to health care providers under Medicare and Medicaid. CMS also administers many provisions of the Affordable Care Act, the 2010 health care reform law often referred to as Obamacare. FDA and CMS are a part of the U.S. Department of Health and Human Services (HHS); DEA is part of the U.S. Department of Justice.

Learning Objectives

Upon completion of this chapter, the reader should be able to:

1. Describe the federal laws and regulations affecting the practice of pharmacy, and name three federal agencies that enforce these requirements.

2. Discuss the history and importance of state boards of pharmacy in the regulation of pharmacists and their professional activities.

3. Compare and contrast pharmacy residencies and pharmacist certification as nongovernmental self-regulation by the profession.

Laws:
Acts passed by a legislative body.

Regulations:
Rules promulgated by a part of the executive branch of government, usually based on a law giving the agency statutory authority for the regulation.

Chapter 7

Misbranded:
Drug products that are not properly labeled as to contents and proper use.

Adulterated:
Products that have been changed or contaminated with impure or foreign substances.

Product labeling:
The information provided with a prescription drug, including the package insert that lists uses, precautions, adverse effects, and dosages of the drug product. The language used in the product labeling must be approved by FDA.

Food and Drug Administration

FDA was created through the passage of the Federal Food and Drugs Act of 1906. In addition to articles in popular magazines and professional journals about the need for federal oversight in this area, two books were important in moving Congress to action: *The Jungle*, by Upton Sinclair, which reviewed atrocities in the meat-packing industry, and *The Great American Fraud*, by Samuel Hopkins Adams, which was a compilation of articles about "patent" medicines.[1] FDA initially had the authority only to pursue manufacturers of already-marketed pharmaceutical products that were **misbranded** or **adulterated.**

In 1937, a terrible tragedy struck the country when a toxic preparation of Elixir Sulfanilamide caused 73 deaths.[1] This resulted in passage of the Food, Drug, and Cosmetic Act of 1938, which expanded FDA's oversight to include premarketing approval of new drug products, medical devices, and cosmetics to determine whether they were safe.[1]

Two important amendments have been made to the 1938 law. In 1952, Congress passed the Durham–Humphrey Amendment, which directed FDA to divide drug products into two categories: those that require a prescription issued by a health care professional authorized to prescribe in the relevant state and those that could be sold without a prescription. In 1962, Congress added more authority by passing the Kefauver–Harris Drug Amendments. These permitted FDA to control research into new drugs, require that new drugs be effective for the conditions listed in **product labeling** (previously, drugs only had to be safe), remove drugs from the market more easily when necessary, and regulate advertising of prescription drugs more easily.[1]

In recent years, FDA's areas of authority have been modified through congressional reviews occurring every 5 years. The fifth such law, the Prescription Drug User Fee Act (PDUFA V), was passed and signed into law in 2012.[2,3] It addressed several areas of current concern. Congress reauthorized FDA user fees through which pharmaceutical manufacturers could pay for expedited review of their products. The fees had become controversial following market withdrawals of some medications in the late 1990s and early 2000s, a period just after the fees were first implemented. The quick approvals combined with market withdrawals of high-profile agents such as Vioxx led some observers to believe the user fees were leading to poor decisions at FDA. But by 2012, several years had passed without another highly publicized market withdrawal, and Congress reauthorized FDA's functioning and funding through user fees.

PDUFA V addressed drug shortages. The pharmaceutical marketplace has become much more centralized and international over the past quarter-century. Some drugs are now made at only a few places worldwide—sometimes even in just one factory. These factories may produce a drug as a powder or other raw pharmaceutical-grade product, or they may produce tablets, capsules, or other dosage forms as required by one or more manufacturers. If natural disasters occur or plants are closed because of quality, financial, or other concerns, the result can be a sudden reduction in the amount of a drug that is available worldwide and a shortage of drug products needed in patient care. PDUFA V requires manufacturers to notify FDA of potential shortages and requires HHS to maintain a list of drugs in short supply.[3]

FDA's system for addressing risks of medications was also addressed in PDUFA V. Over the years, FDA had made many different requirements of manufacturers when drug products offered benefits to patients but also caused adverse effects in some or all patients that needed to be addressed or watched for. These were termed *risk evaluation and mitigation strategies*, or REMS. As the number of drug products with REMS grew, pharmacists and other health care professionals found it difficult to determine what the precise requirements were for each product. PDUFA V gave FDA statutory authority to address this problem through a REMS Integration Initiative. The intent is for FDA to standardize REMS and look for routine ways of assessing their impact.[2] The new law also called for FDA to use biomarkers and pharmacogenomics in developing REMS for drug products used in serious diseases.[3]

FDA regulation of dietary supplements—which include herbal products, vitamins/minerals, and natural products such as fish oils and glucosamine/chondroitin—was problematic for many decades after drug product regulations became routine. The Dietary Supplement Health and Education Act of 1994 (DSHEA) permitted "structure/function claims" to be made for dietary supplements without proof of safety or efficacy by the manufacturer or distributor. This, in effect, means that FDA must prove a product to be useless or harmful to remove it from the market. This is the exact opposite of the system under which drug products are approved in that the burden of proof of safety and effectiveness for prescription and over-the-counter drugs lies with the manufacturer and FDA rules on these claims before marketing.[4]

FDA in 2000 issued regulations clarifying what is a permitted structure/function claim under DSHEA and what in its view constitutes an unacceptable "disease claim" for dietary supplements.[4] FDA included as structure/function claims effects on common conditions associated with aging, pregnancy, menopause, and adolescence. Conditions that many consumers and professionals view as diseases—such as morning sickness and premenstrual syndrome (PMS)—are now permissible structure/function claims. Thus, labels of dietary supplements might include language such as the following:
- For common symptoms of PMS
- For hot flashes

FDA also allows dietary supplements to contain "health maintenance" claims, such as
- Maintains a healthy circulatory system
- For muscle enhancement
- Helps you relax

Express disease claims ("prevents osteoporosis," "prevents bone fragility in postmenopausal women") remain forbidden. However, some structure/function claims (such as "prevents memory loss") will undoubtedly lead some patients and caregivers to believe the products can be used for treating diseases where those claims are relevant (in that case, improving cognition in Alzheimer's disease).

Following the 2003 death of a Baltimore Orioles pitcher who was taking the dietary supplement ephedra, the pendulum began swinging back to tighter regulation of the supplements industry.[5] In 2007, FDA published final regulations that tightened quality control over dietary supplements,[4] and these should decrease problems with what had been a perpetual source of uncertainty regarding use of these products.

"Any movement contains the seeds of its own destruction. Gradually they may grow until the movement itself is overshadowed, until its originators find themselves in the uncomfortable position of condoning what they had condemned, and of following what they had organized to oppose. Thus, too, in pharmacy. Some organizations dedicated to avoiding legal restrictions became the initiators and, subsequently, the guardians of American pharmaceutical legislation."

—Glenn Sonnedecker, in Kremers and Urdang's *History of Pharmacy*, fourth edition, page 213

A perpetual issue at FDA is a proposed third class of drugs that could be prescribed and dispensed by pharmacists. The term *third class* comes from the fact that drugs are currently divided into two classes: those that require a prescriber's prescription and those that can be sold over the counter (OTC) with no health care professional involved. Opponents of such behind-the-counter (BTC) medications include physician groups and a trade association that represents companies that sell OTC medicines.

Drug Enforcement Administration

DEA is responsible for the regulation of controlled substances in the United States. Controlled substances are those with abuse and addiction potential. DEA was created in 1970 by the Comprehensive Drug Abuse Prevention and Control Act and the Controlled Substances Act.[7]

Federal law divides controlled substances into five schedules that have different requirements for handling and record keeping:

- *Schedule I.* These drugs have high abuse and addiction potential and no accepted medical use in the United States. Examples are heroin, LSD, marijuana, and mescaline.
- *Schedule II.* These drugs have high abuse and addiction potential but do have medical applications. Examples include cocaine, Dilaudid (hydromorphone), Ritalin (methylphenidate), Seconal (secobarbital), and several types of amphetamines ("diet pills" or "speed").
- *Schedule III.* These drugs have abuse and addiction potential but not as much as those in Schedule II. Examples are Tylenol #3 (acetaminophen with codeine) and Fastin (phentermine).
- *Schedule IV.* These drugs have a low potential for abuse. Examples include Valium (diazepam), Halcion (triazolam), and Darvon (dextropropoxyphene).
- *Schedule V.* Drugs in this schedule have low abuse potential and have very limited amounts of drugs in each dosage form. Examples are Lomotil (diphenoxylate and atropine) and some cough syrups containing codeine. Some Schedule V products do not require a prescription (through FDA regulations), but they must be dispensed by a pharmacist because of DEA rules.

DEA today has many responsibilities for fighting the illicit drug trafficking problem, and pharmacy is only a small part of this job. DEA agents thus have two different roles, one in which they fight criminals who are smuggling and selling huge quantities of illegal drugs and another in which they must apprehend health care professionals who are diverting legal drugs into the illegal market. Different divisions of DEA work in these two areas, but many pharmacists think that DEA agents act inappropriately when they deal with health care professionals.

Centers for Medicare & Medicaid Services

CMS is the current name for the agency that administers federal coverage of health care. It was known as the Health Care Financing Administration from its inception during the Great Society phase of the Johnson administration in 1965 until it was renamed during the Bush administration in 2001. This agency is responsible for implementation and administration of the Affordable Care Act.[8]

While the Medicare and Medicaid programs are very complicated, one can think of the Medicare program as paying for acute (hospital) care for the elderly and the Medicaid program as covering the **indigent**. Until 2006, Medicare paid for prescription drugs only when they were used in an acute care institution (hospital) or in conjunction with certain medical devices such as in-dwelling catheters (tubes that go into very large veins of the body). Beginning in 2006, Part D coverage was added to Medicare to pay for prescription drugs. Medicaid pays for outpatient prescription drugs and other care for indigent patients in community pharmacies, nursing homes, or hospitals. Some people qualify for both Medicare and Medicaid, and they are termed *dual eligibles*.

Important to note is that the Medicaid program is financed jointly by the federal and state governments, with each contributing about one-half of the funds. Thus, although Medicaid is a federal program, pharmacists' interactions are usually with the agency within their state government that coordinates the program. As state budgets have been squeezed more and more recently, the Medicaid programs have been increasingly tightened. The effects of these economic constraints have been severe in many states. For example, Medicaid patients' prescriptions often must be filled using a state-approved drug list (or formulary), recipients may be limited to a certain number of prescriptions per month, and states have sometimes held up Medicaid payments for several months because of budgetary shortfall.

The Affordable Care Act added another layer of complexity to Medicaid. In states that accepted an expanded Medicaid program under the law, the federal government initially paid 100% of the costs of these new Medicaid enrollees. This figure will decline to 90% of costs by 2020.

Medicare Part D is a federal program, but it is administered through dozens of private prescription drug providers, or PDPs. Each PDP has its own formulary, and Medicare beneficiaries can choose any PDP operating in their geographic area (usually a state). Pharmacists' interactions are generally with these intermediaries when it comes to obtaining reimbursement for prescriptions and getting approval for nonformulary medications.

As mentioned in Chapter 3, Medicare Part D includes a provision for medication therapy management (MTM) services. PDPs are required to provide, either directly or through other entities (such as pharmacies), MTM services to Medicare patients who are being treated for multiple diseases with multiple medications and who are expected to need medications costing several thousand dollars during the year. CMS has stated that MTM services should become the cornerstone of Medicare Part D, and the associated payment aspect could enable pharmacists to further develop their pharmaceutical care and clinical pharmacy services for older patients. If this happens, the pharmacist's role in processing and preparing prescription medications will become even more important than it is today.

In addition to the daily requirements associated with processing individual prescriptions, pharmacies must comply with certain broader requirements mandated by CMS and/or state agencies. These are called *conditions of participation* because providers—including hospitals, physicians, nursing homes, and pharmacies—must agree to them in

Indigent:
Unable to pay for certain basic services for oneself, including health care.

Class of trade:
Customers of a business or industry may be divided into one or more groups based on their purchasing and payment characteristics. Each of these classes of trade is dealt with differently — and may receive different prices or payment policies — because of the interplay between these characteristics and the sellers' goals and objectives relative to that part of the industry.

order to participate in the Medicare and Medicaid programs. Conditions for participation specify many operational, procedural, and outcome details, and you may see that your pharmacy is changing a procedure or getting new equipment for making intravenous fluids because of such requirements.

Serious problems with Medicare and Medicaid fraud continue to crop up for pharmacists and other health care providers. With spending for these programs above $1 trillion annually, the possibilities for substantial amounts of fraud are quite high.

In 1990, Congress passed a bill that directed the Health Care Financing Administration (now CMS) to begin collecting rebates from pharmaceutical manufacturers based on the difference between the manufacturers' best price to any buyer of that product and the price of that drug to the government under the Medicaid program of the state. This has caused manufacturers to reassess their basic pricing structures, with detrimental results for hospitals and other institutions with nonprofit or government status. Beginning during World War II, manufacturers had created a separate **class of trade** for nonprofit and government buyers of their products, and prices for this group were sometimes only a small fraction of the price paid by community pharmacies. This gave the nonprofit/government institutions an unfair competitive advantage. Under current Medicaid provisions, manufacturers are encouraged to eliminate this price differential; if they do not, the Medicaid program benefits by obtaining rebates from the manufacturers for products dispensed through community pharmacies at Medicaid expense.

State laws and regulations

Agencies of the state government are very important to pharmacists. Since the people in these agencies are much closer geographically to the pharmacy, the possibilities for frequent contacts are that much higher.

State boards of pharmacy

The division of responsibilities between the state and federal governments follows the line of reasoning known as states' rights: All responsibilities not specifically assigned to the federal government in the U.S. Constitution are reserved for the states. The area of drug and pharmacy regulation has been one in which the federal government has creatively enlarged its role when it thought that the public health was at risk, but the states remain an integral part of the regulatory framework.

The mechanism by which states regulate professions is through boards composed largely of members of a given profession along with one or two consumer members. Federal laws generally do not deal specifically with regulation of professions; for instance, FDA's legend drugs do not specify what types of practitioners may legally prescribe these drugs. Federal law thus depends heavily on the framework that states put in place during the last half of the nineteenth century.

State boards of pharmacy developed around 1900 after their organization had been proposed in model pharmacy laws developed by the American Pharmaceutical (now Pharmacists) Association. As Sonnedecker has described so well, pharmacy organizations and pharmacy laws have often grown together, and the organization of state pharmacy boards followed this trend.[1] However, it is important to remember that state boards of pharmacy have as their primary mission the protection of the public from the profession—not vice versa. Pharmacy associations, conversely, exist to promote the profession, which sometimes leads them along paths that are not necessarily in the best interests of the public.

State boards of pharmacy, based on authority granted to them by the various state legislatures, promulgate the specific regulations that govern the practice of pharmacy on a day-to-day basis. Boards issue **licenses** to pharmacists and pharmacies, specify by what mechanisms pharmacists can keep their licenses in force, have investigative arms that police the profession, and are the judge and jury for pharmacists who violate state pharmacy laws. For the student pharmacist, learning state pharmacy laws and preparing for the board of pharmacy examinations are major foci of activity. For the practicing pharmacist, the decisions rendered by a state board of pharmacy can drastically affect the way in which the profession must be practiced in that state.

In 1904, a national organization of state boards of pharmacy was formed.[1] The National Association of Boards of Pharmacy (NABP) has grown to a powerful position in coordinating activities among the state boards. It now provides a national examination, called NAPLEX, for North American Pharmacist Licensure Examination, for administration in all states. NABP coordinates the **reciprocation** of pharmacist licenses across states. The association develops model pharmacy practice acts that state legislatures can consider in updating state laws to incorporate changes in pharmacy.

Other state agencies

At the state level, the other primary agency of concern to pharmacists is the one that handles the Medicaid program. Because these agencies vary greatly by state, it is not possible to provide a uniform description, but you can talk with pharmacists in your state about what your agency is like. Also, inquire about pharmacy faculty at your school who may work with the state agency in analyzing drug-use trends.

Most states have some type of controlled-substances counterpart to DEA, and pharmacists interface with those agencies as well.

Self-governance by pharmacy

Increasingly important in pharmacy is the process of **accreditation** of residency and training programs and **certification** of individual practitioners for increased knowledge in pharmacy specialty areas. As opposed to the mandatory licensure described for pharmacists, accreditation and certification are examples of voluntary oversight by the profession. Let's look at how they work.

Accreditation of training programs

Most people are familiar with the process by which physicians enter residency programs to specialize in various medical areas. But not many members of the public real-

License:
A document issued to pharmacists and other citizens that provides special privileges based on specialized knowledge or skills. A driver's license is one type of such document; it permits the holder to operate motorized vehicles on public roads based on a demonstration to the state of sufficient knowledge. A pharmacy license permits the holder to engage in a specialized profession known as pharmacy following demonstration to the state of adequate knowledge. It is a privilege, not a right, and thus the state may withdraw the privilege for various reasons.

Reciprocation:
Once a pharmacist is licensed, he or she can use that license (if in good standing) to practice in other states, after the state board of pharmacy in the new state recognizes the license from the previous state.

Accreditation:
Recognition of a residency or other type of program by comparing it with standards set by the accrediting body. This standard describes the goals or ideals that each program should strive for and sets certain minimum criteria that each should maintain.

Certification:
Recognition of an individual for specialized knowledge or skills based on demonstration of that knowledge or those skills to the certifying body. The term certification carries the connotation that the certifying body is a non-government entity, and the recognition typically carries no legally defined privileges.

ize that many pharmacy graduates enter residency programs; as the entry-level PharmD movement has taken hold, an increasing number of graduates are going on for this type of specialized training.

Pharmacy residencies developed first in hospital pharmacy in the 1930s (they were called *internships* until 1962), and residencies in hospitals are still the most common type. The American Society of Hospital (now Health-System) Pharmacists (ASHP) began accrediting hospital pharmacy residencies in 1963, and it currently recognizes more than 2,000 programs. ASHP eliminated its hospital pharmacy and clinical pharmacy residencies in 1992; all are now recognized as pharmacy residencies. ASHP also offers several types of specialized residencies (see Chapter 10), and in 1999 it began accrediting managed care and community pharmacy residencies with, respectively, the Academy of Managed Care Pharmacy and the American Pharmaceutical (now Pharmacists) Association.[9]

In 2003, the ASHP reorganized its accreditation standards into postgraduate year 1 (PGY1) and postgraduate year 2 (PGY2). PGY1 programs can be conducted at one or more sites, and colleges of pharmacy can participate as sponsoring organizations. Residents learn about managing and improving the medication-use process; providing evidence-based, patient-centered medication therapy management with interdisciplinary teams; exercising leadership and practice management skills; demonstrating project management skills; providing medication and practice-related education/training; and using medical informatics.[9] PGY2 pharmacy residency programs focus on a specific area of practice, such as primary care/ambulatory care, critical care, drug information, geriatrics, oncology, psychiatric, or internal medicine.[10]

In 2014, ASHP and the Accreditation Council for Pharmacy Education formed the Pharmacy Technician Accreditation Commission, which accredits pharmacy technician training programs. Accredited programs are based chiefly in community colleges and technical schools, but some hospitals and colleges of pharmacy also have such programs. In 2013, ASHP had 258 programs in the accreditation process.[11]

Certification of individuals

Certification is a term that is becoming increasingly common in pharmacy, particularly in two areas: for pharmacists who practice in highly specialized areas and for pharmacy technicians. Certification is a form of self-discipline or self-control by a profession, and the process works when employers and health care professionals are able to police themselves. For instance, any physician can legally perform brain surgery, but only those who are certified by a medical specialty board as neurosurgeons generally do so. But if a substantial number of noncertified physicians began offering services they were not qualified to perform and the public was at risk of harm as a result, the state would likely step in and set up a licensure mechanism.

In pharmacy, the Board of Pharmacy Specialties (BPS) was organized in 1975 to recognize what activities in pharmacy required certification and to develop processes to accomplish that certification. Since then, it has recognized nearly 25,000 pharmacists in eight specialties:[12]

- Ambulatory care pharmacy
- Critical care pharmacy
- Nuclear pharmacy
- Nutrition support pharmacy
- Oncology pharmacy
- Pediatric pharmacy
- Pharmacotherapy
- Psychiatric pharmacy

In addition, infectious diseases and cardiology are recognized as areas of added qualifications under the pharmacotherapy specialty. This means that board-certified pharmacotherapists who practice primarily in infectious diseases or cardiology can be recognized.

The purpose of pharmacy certification is to demonstrate personal achievement in these specialized areas. Employers also often require applicants to have certain credentials, including certification status in one of these specialty areas.

For an area to be recognized by BPS as a specialty, one or more sponsoring organizations must submit a detailed petition outlining the specialty and related details. If approved as a specialty by BPS, the sponsoring organizations then participate in development of a certification examination that is given once or twice a year. Those attaining a certain score on the exam are designated as certified and are eligible to use certain initials after their names.

Pharmacy technicians are also becoming certified. For them, certification is a way to demonstrate accomplishment in a career that has no uniform education or training requirements and to show employers a given level of knowledge about the activities of pharmacy technicians. The Pharmacy Technician Certification Board is the certifying body for pharmacy technicians, and it had certified nearly 600,000 pharmacy technicians at the end of 2015,[13] more than the number of licensed pharmacists in the United States.

Employers use certification of technicians as a way of determining promotions into jobs such as those in intravenous admixture rooms or supervising other technicians.

Overregulated and loving it

As this chapter shows, pharmacy is definitely a well-regulated profession. But interestingly, pharmacists often lobby for more regulation when they want to move the profession in a certain direction. For instance, nothing made much difference in pharmacists' interest in patient counseling until national pharmacy groups caused Congress to mandate it for Medicaid recipients. For some reason, pharmacy has had more success with having the government keep the playing field level than it has with stimulating its members to raise their own professional sights. Pharmacists indeed have become the initiators and the guardians of those laws that specify sometimes very precisely what pharmacists must and must not do.

REFERENCES

1. Sonnedecker G. The rise of legislative standards. In: *Kremers and Urdang's History of Pharmacy.* 4th ed. Philadelphia, Pa.: Lippincott; 1976:213–25.

2. PDUFA V: Fiscal years 2013–2017. U.S. Food and Drug Administration Web site. www.fda.gov/ForIndustry/UserFees/PrescriptionDrugUserFee/ucm272170.htm. Accessed June 6, 2016.

3. Yap D. PDUFA V becomes law. *Pharm Today.* 2012;18(8):62.

4. Dietary supplements. U.S. Food and Drug Administration Web site. www.fda.gov/Food/DietarySupplements/. Accessed June 6, 2016.

5. Posey LM. FDA moves on dietary supplement quality, ephedra safety. *Pharm Today.* 2003;9(4):1, 4.

6. Monastersky N, Landau SC. Future of emergency contraception lies in pharmacists' hands. *J Am Pharm Assoc.* 2006;46(1):84–8.

7. DEA history. U.S. Drug Enforcement Administration Web site. www.dea.gov/about/history.shtml. Accessed June 6, 2016.

8. CMS' program history. Centers for Medicare & Medicaid Services Web site. www.cms.gov/About-CMS/Agency-Information/History/. Accessed June 6, 2016.

9. Residency program directors. American Society of Health-System Pharmacists Web site. www.ashp.org/menu/Residency/Residency-Program-Directors. Accessed June 6, 2016.

10. Accreditation standards for PGY1 pharmacy residencies. American Society of Health-System Pharmacists Web site. www.ashp.org/menu/Residency/Residency-Program-Directors/Accreditation-Standards-for-PGY1-Pharmacy-Residencies.aspx. Accessed June 6, 2016.

11. Pharmacy Technician Accreditation Commission (PTAC). American Society of Health-System Pharmacists Web site. www.ashp.org/menu/Technicians/Technician-Accreditation/PTAC.aspx. Accessed June 6, 2016.

12. Board of Pharmacy Specialties Web site. www.bpsweb.org. Accessed June 6, 2016.

13. Pharmacy Technician Certification Board Web site. www.ptcb.org. Accessed June 6, 2016.

Chapter 8 | Pharmacy Associations: Opportunities for Pharmacists and Student Pharmacists

Abir A. (Abby) Kahaleh

Most major national pharmacy associations have been mentioned somewhere in Chapters 1-7 of this textbook, but a brief, straightforward presentation of material is always useful. In this chapter, I provide information about the major pharmacy practitioner organizations and their histories, current status, strengths, weaknesses, and relationships with each other.

A consortium of national pharmacy practitioner organizations, the Joint Commission of Pharmacy Practitioners, was founded in 1977, and it meets quarterly in Washington, D.C. The members are listed in Table 8.1, along with contact information, and these are the primary organizations that I discuss in this chapter.

JCPP has been an extremely effective tool for bringing to one table the leaders of American pharmacy from all sectors of the profession. People are sometimes disappointed that JCPP does not take more of an activist role, but that is not the nature of consortia. The group works through consensus building, not motions and votes. If even one member of JCPP cannot agree on a course of action about an issue, generally no action is taken, and this leaves the individual associations free to pursue their own agendas in their own ways. However, many positive joint statements, alliances, and unified actions have been facilitated because of the meetings of JCPP.

Recently, JCPP approved the Pharmacists' Patient Care Process. Specifically, the JCPP indicated that "Patients will achieve optimal health and medication outcomes when pharmacists are included as essential and accountable members of patient-centered healthcare teams."[1] Several other non-JCPP organizations also form an important part of the framework within which pharmacists operate. These are listed in Table 8.2 with brief descriptions of the focus of each.

The Accreditation Council for Pharmacy Education (ACPE) includes activities to optimize pharmacy education and advance pharmacy practice.[2] Specifically, co-curricular activities have been defined in the 2016 Standards as student involvement in didactic and experiential education to complement, augment, and enhance students' competencies.[2] Co-curricular experiences can be developed by student professional organizations or external groups, including local or regional pharmacy associations.

At the American Pharmacists Association (APhA), the Academy of Student Pharmacists (APhA–ASP) has local chapters at all the colleges and schools of pharmacy. APhA–ASP hosts Midyear Regional Meetings designated for student pharmacists across the United States.[3] These meetings offer opportunities for leadership development, advocacy initiatives, networking, and community outreach programs.

Learning Objectives

Upon completion of this chapter, the reader should be able to:

1. Identify professional development opportunities for pharmacists and student pharmacists at pharmacy associations.

2. Develop professional networks with colleagues and mentors with similar aspiring career goals.

3. Compare and contrast professional opportunities at various pharmacy associations.

With that background, here are descriptions of the pharmacy practitioner organizations that are in the JCPP.

Table 8.1 | Members of the Joint Commission of Pharmacy Practitioners

Organizations	Year Founded	Number of Staff	Budget ($, Millions)	No. People (at Largest Meeting)	Number of Members	Student Dues ($)	Web Address
Regular JCPP members							
APhA (American Pharmacists Association)	1852	120	34	7,000	60,000	45	www.pharmacist.com
NCPA (National Community Pharmacists Association)	1898	200	35	3,000	22,000	50	www.ncpanet.org
ACA (American College of Apothecaries)	1940	6	0.4	200	1,000	Free	www.acainfo.org
AMCP (Academy of Managed Care Pharmacy)	1989	30	1	3,000	8,000	45	www.amcp.org
ASHP (American Society of Health-System Pharmacists)	1942	170	43	20,000	43,000	49	www.ashp.org
ASCP (American Society of Consultant Pharmacists)	1968	39	5	1,000	9,000	Free (1 yr.) 80 (Graduate)	www.ascp.com
ACCP (American College of Clinical Pharmacy)	1979	18	4	2,149	15,000	40	www.accp.com
Affiliate members[a]							
NABP (National Association of Boards of Pharmacy)	1904	32	5.0	550	66[b] (54 active/ 12 associate)	N.A.	www.nabp.net
NASPA (National Alliance of State Pharmacy Associations)	~1930	3	0.065	50	51[c] (76 associate)	N.A.	www.naspa.us
AACP (American Association of Colleges of Pharmacy)	1900	21	13	2,309	[d]	15	www.aacp.org 703/739-2330
ACPE[e] (Accreditation Council for Pharmacy Education)	1932	13	4	N.A.	N.A.	N.A.	www.acpe-accredit.org 312/664-3575

Source: Adapted from information provided by Dr. Joseph A. Oddis, former executive vice president of the American Society of Health-System Pharmacists.

[a] Because these groups are not pharmacy practitioner organizations, they are not discussed in detail in this chapter.

[b] As was mentioned in Chapter 7, NABP is the organization representing the state boards of pharmacy. Headquartered in suburban Chicago, NABP conducts an annual meeting for members of the state boards, prepares documents such as model pharmacy practice acts that increase consistency in pharmacy laws from state to state, and participates in committees and consortia that work on pharmacy-practice issues related to state pharmacy law (see Chapter 7).

[c] NASPA is a group representing staff members who head state pharmacy associations. Currently, one statewide pharmacy association from each state is permitted to have a member in NASPA; this member is from the umbrella pharmacy organization (versus the state group of health-system, consultant, or clinical pharmacists).

[d] AACP is a combination individual and trade association representing the interests of the administration and faculties of colleges of pharmacy and individual members. It publishes a journal, conducts an annual meeting, and participates in many ways in dialogues within the pharmacy community about pharmacy practice roles and how they relate to pharmacy education and research.

[e] ACPE is the accrediting body for pharmacy schools and providers of pharmaceutical continuing education. Funds come from fees charged to pharmacy schools and CPE providers; membership on the board of directors is appointed by APhA, AACP, and other pharmacy associations.

Table 8.2 | Other Pharmacy-Related Associations

Association	Description
American Association of Pharmaceutical Scientists (AAPS) 703-243-2800 www.aaps.org	An individual membership organization representing researchers in the pharmaceutical sciences; founded as a spinoff organization from APhA during the 1980s.
American Foundation for Pharmaceutical Education (AFPE) 301-738-2160 www.afpenet.org	Uses grants from industry and other sources to fund scholarships, fellowships, and other grants for pharmacy students at the undergraduate and postgraduate levels.
American Institute of the History of Pharmacy (AIHP) 608-262-5378 www.pharmacy.wisc.edu/aihp	An institute devoted to the study and preservation of the history of pharmacy.
Consumer Healthcare Products Association (CHPA) 202-429-9260 www.chpa-info.org	A trade association representing the interests of companies that manufacture and distribute nonprescription drugs. Often in conflict with pharmacy associations, especially on the "third class of drugs" issue.
Healthcare Distribution Management Association 703-787-0000 www.healthcaredistribution.org	A trade association representing wholesale druggists and other organizations that serve as the "middle men" in the health care product distribution chain.
International Pharmaceutical Federation (FIP) +31-70-3021970 www.fip.org	An international association of pharmacists. Holds an annual session the first week in September. Some information about FIP available from APhA and ASHP.
National Association of Chain Drug Stores (NACDS) 703-549-3001 www.nacds.org	A trade association of nearly 200 chain drug stores that operate 37,000 pharmacies. Conducts an annual meeting, a pharmaceutical conference, and other meetings each year. Very involved in governmental tracking and lobbying at the national and state levels. Publishes various newsletters and informational alerts for its members.
National Council on Patient Information and Education (NCPIE) 301-656-8565 www.talkaboutrx.org	A privately funded organization that conducts national campaigns to educate consumers about the drugs they take and that encourages pharmacists and other health care providers to provide more information to consumers. Sponsors "Talk About Prescriptions" month each October.
National Pharmaceutical Council (NPC) 703-620-6390 www.npcnow.org	A trade association that conducts public relations activities on behalf of major research-oriented pharmaceutical firms.
Pharmaceutical Care Management Association (PCMA) 202-207-3610 www.pcmanet.org	A trade association representing companies that provide pharmacy benefit managers, including mail-service pharmacies.
Pharmaceutical Research and Manufacturers of America (PhRMA) 202-835-3400 www.phrma.org	A trade association representing the research-oriented pharmaceutical industry. Heavily involved in lobbying at the state and federal levels.
Poison Prevention Week Council 301/504-7058 www.poisonprevention.org	The organization that coordinates Poison Prevention Week activities during the third week of March each year.
Pharmacy Quality Alliance (PQA) 703-690-1987 www.PQAAlliance.org	A pharmacy quality alliance, PQA is a collaborative initiative that seeks to define quality measures for pharmacist and pharmacy services.
United States Pharmacopeial Convention 301/881-0666 www.usp.org	The national body that sets standards for drug products in the United States. Has quasi-governmental status because its pronouncements on drug quality, assay methodology, and standards have the weight of federal law.

"It is my firm conviction that American pharmacy will not come into its own until we have a majority of our pharmacists actively supporting their national professional organization. Someone has defined an organization as a medium for the efficient movement of groups of men towards goals to which they aspire. How can we move American pharmacists towards professional goals until we enroll them in our Association? Only when this is done will the Association, its ideals, its ethics, its concepts of professional service become ingrained in all who practice our profession."

—Donald E. Francke, in his 1953 Harvey A. K. Whitney Lecture Award Address

American Pharmacists Association

Formed in 1852 as the American Pharmaceutical Association, the American Pharmacists Association is the oldest and largest organization in pharmacy. It occupies a prominent position in the nation's capital, both politically and geographically: APhA is the organization that Congress expects to speak for pharmacy, and its historic building—with a new annex now under construction—on Constitution Avenue across from the Vietnam Veterans Memorial and Lincoln Memorial is the only private structure on that impressive boulevard.

Today's APhA is a strong organization, one that is positioned well to help pharmacists incorporate medication therapy management (MTM) into their practices. APhA uses these vision, mission, and tagline statements to guide its programs and services:

- *APhA's Vision for Society:* Pharmacists and patients working together to improve medication use and health.
- *APhA's Mission:* The American Pharmacists Association provides information, education and advocacy to help all pharmacists improve medication use and advance patient care.
- *APhA's Tagline:* The American Pharmacists Association. Improving Medication Use. Advancing Patient Care.

APhA has more than 60,000 members (including practicing pharmacists, pharmaceutical scientists, student pharmacists, pharmacy technicians, and others interested in advancing the profession) and strong assets. As the only national organization that can claim to represent all of pharmacy, its pronouncements are respected and its activities noticed.

Members of APhA include some 30,000 members of APhA–ASP. It also has strong, influential membership segments of pharmacy school faculty, pharmacists who work for the federal government (e.g., in the military or the U.S. Public Health Service or for the Department of Veterans Affairs), hospital pharmacists, and community pharmacists. Membership in APhA's House of Delegates is determined by state pharmacists associations, giving a voice to pharmacists politically active at the state level. APhA seeks to represent the interests of employee pharmacists in all settings, and it has been successful in developing this concept through a new practitioner program. The idea has a lot of potential for future expansions of APhA membership, since the nation's community chain pharmacists are basically unrepresented in national pharmacy organizations.

The APhA Annual Meeting and Exposition, which includes the annual meeting of ASP, is held during the spring. Sites are rotated among the various large cities in the United States and sometimes Canada. Upward of 2,500 student pharmacists attend the APhA annual meeting each year. In the fall, APhA–ASP's Midyear Regional Meetings are held in the group's eight regions.

Publications are an important part of APhA's services and budget. In addition to its monthly pharmacist patient care services magazine, *Pharmacy Today*; drug information newsletter, *APhA DrugInfoLine*; and journals, *Journal of the American Pharmacists Association* and *Journal of Pharmaceutical Sciences*, APhA publishes a number of books, including the important titles *Handbook of Nonprescription Drugs* and *Medication Errors*. APhA also publishes a daily summary of news relevant to pharmacists, the daily edition of *Pharmacy Today*.

APhA's website, www.pharmacist.com, offers breaking news coverage, news articles from *Pharmacy Today* and the *APhA DrugInfoLine,* legislative and regulatory updates, continuing education, and resource centers for emerging practice trends such as MTM. Many parts of the site are available to everyone, whereas other pages are for APhA members only.

In the professional arena, APhA is quite involved in setting policy and standards of practice for pharmacy in all settings. Through its House of Delegates, many important policies express the pharmacy profession's viewpoints on controversial issues such as assisted suicide and ethics for pharmacists. These policies are communicated to other associations and policy makers in the federal and state governments by APhA's growing staff, which stands currently at 135 employees.

MTM and patient care services in all settings, but especially in community independent and chain pharmacies, have been areas of particular emphasis for APhA over the past several years. Its foundation, a separate organization, has sponsored or been involved in Project ImPACT and the Asheville Project, both demonstration projects showing that pharmacists who meet one-on-one with patients with chronic diseases (e.g., diabetes, hypertension, dyslipidemias, depression, asthma) can make a tremendous difference in clinical, financial, and quality-of-life outcomes.

On the practice front, APhA has been a leader in gaining recognition of pharmacists as health care providers. As mentioned in Chapter 6, this initiative targeted the three main strategic goals:
- Improve access, quality, and value of health care.
- Ensure access and coverage for pharmacists' patient care services through Medicare, Medicaid, integrated care delivery systems, and private payers.
- Include pharmacists as members of interprofessional health care teams.

On the educational front, the APhA–ASP National Patient Care and Community Service Projects provide opportunities for student pharmacists to engage in co-curricular experiences in various health care and community outreach programs. Specifically, these programs include Generation Rx, Operation Diabetes, Operation Heart, Operation Immunization, and OTC Medicine Safety. Additional information on each program can be found at the APhA–ASP web page at www.pharmacist.com.

APhA also serves as a home for two other important parts of the profession: the Board of Pharmacy Specialties (BPS) and the Pharmacy Technician Certification Board (PTCB). BPS (www.bpsweb.org), as described in Chapter 7, certifies pharmacists at the advanced practice specialty level in numerous specialties. PTCB (www.ptcb.org), described in Chapter 7, is a separate organization that certifies pharmacy technicians.

As American society has grown more diverse, many large national associations that represent broad but splintering fields have encountered difficulties in being all things to all members. APhA is no exception. At times, in trying to meet the needs of all parts of the profession, APhA finds various subcomponents of its diverse membership in conflict with one another. More narrowly focused pharmacy organizations have sometimes pulled members away from APhA, leaving it with fewer resources to respond to problems, opportunities, and crises for the profession.

Important for pharmacists to remember is that we are all in the same boat—we will float together or we will sink together. For more than a century and a half, APhA has been our boat.

American Society of Health-System Pharmacists

The American Society of Health-System Pharmacists (ASHP) is the national professional society for pharmacists who practice in hospitals and health systems. Founded as the American Society of Hospital Pharmacists in 1942, the society's 40,000 members include pharmacists who practice in inpatient, ambulatory, home care, and long-term-care settings, as well as pharmacy technicians and student pharmacists.

ASHP's mission is to "help people achieve optimal health outcomes." As part of that mission, ASHP strives to advocate and support "the professional practice of pharmacists in hospitals, health systems, ambulatory clinics, and other settings spanning the full spectrum of medication use" and to serve "its members as their collective voice on issues related to medication use and public health."

ASHP began its life in 1936 as a subsection of hospital pharmacists at APhA. Officially founded in 1942, the society became fully autonomous in 1960 when it opened its first full-time office in Washington, D.C., and hired Joseph A. Oddis, ScD, as executive vice president. ASHP moved to Bethesda, Maryland, in 1966 and has been located in that Washington, D.C., suburb ever since. In 1994, ASHP changed to its current name to reflect the changes occurring in the hospital industry as many hospitals began linking as systems and diversifying beyond inpatient care, as well as to recognize that many ASHP members serve patients in outpatient clinics and home care operations associated with hospitals.

Started with an initial group of 154 charter members, the organization has grown to more than 40,000 members. As an organization focused on serving pharmacists who practice in hospitals and health systems, the society offers membership sections that provide tailored resources to pharmacists in specific areas of practice. The following member sections and forums serve as a "home within a home" for members who provide input on the society's policy-making process, educational resources, and other programs:
• Section of Ambulatory Care Practitioners
• Section of Clinical Specialists and Scientists
• Section of Inpatient Care Practitioners
• Section of Pharmacy Informatics and Technology
• Section of Pharmacy Practice Managers

The society also provides two membership forums—the Student Forum and the New Practitioner's Forum—for pharmacists just starting their careers. The forums offer resources across practice settings that can help students and new practitioners gain insights from their pharmacy peers and provide leadership opportunities.

The society maintains affiliate relationships with state-based health-system pharmacy organizations throughout the United States. ASHP is aligned with student societies of health-system pharmacy at nearly all colleges and schools of pharmacy.

Other areas of emphasis for ASHP include accreditation of pharmacy residency and technician-training programs; publishing journals and books (including the respected reference text, *AHFS Drug Information*); providing practitioner education; advocacy at the federal and state levels; public relations; a research and education foundation; and maintenance of a dynamic website.

Throughout its history, ASHP has been driven by the ideals of improving patient safety and advancing the practice of pharmacy in hospitals and health systems. Steadfast devotion to these ideals have allowed ASHP to effect practice change and provide pharmacists in hospitals and health systems with the tools they need to best care for their patients.

The Student Society of Health-System Pharmacy (SSHP) has several chapters nationwide. Each SSHP is recognized by ASHP and has an affiliation with the ASHP state association.[4] To become an "officially" recognized SSHP, the society must have programming that is consistent with mission of ASHP, meet the annual requirements, and educate members about career options in hospitals and health systems.

ASHP–SSHP recognition criteria include the following:[4]
1. Career development:
   - Clinical skills competition
   - Pharmacy speakers
   - Residency and training information session
2. Professional development: Project directly related to the ASHP Strategic Plan
3. Membership recruitment: Membership drive (SSHP–State Affiliate–ASHP)

American College of Clinical Pharmacy

Founded in 1979 by ASHP members who practiced clinical pharmacy at an advanced level, the American College of Clinical Pharmacy (ACCP) is another rapidly growing pharmacy association. Like the American College of Apothecaries (ACA), the college's criteria for full membership are more restrictive than those of other pharmacy organizations; in these criteria, ACCP emphasizes experience in practicing or teaching patient-oriented clinical pharmacy.

ACCP's mission is "to advance human health by extending the frontiers of clinical pharmacy. Through strategic initiatives, partnerships, collaborations, and alliances, ACCP:
- Provides leadership, professional development, advocacy, and resources that enable clinical pharmacists to achieve excellence in practice, research, and education.
- Advances clinical pharmacy and pharmacotherapy through support and promotion of research, training, and education.
- Promotes innovative science, develops successful models of practice, and disseminates new knowledge to advance pharmacotherapy and patient care."[5]

With a membership of 15,000, ACCP has gone through several phases during its brief history. Until 1986, ACCP was closely aligned with the journal *Drug Intelligence & Clinical Pharmacy* (known today as *Annals of Pharmacotherapy*), which served as its offices and provided some staff support. Since 1986, ACCP has had paid staff based in the Kansas City, Missouri, area, and has named the journal *Pharmacotherapy* as its official publication. ACCP established a Washington, D.C., office in 2000, through which the college pursues an advocacy agenda set annually by its Board of Regents.

Tertiary-care institutions: Hospitals that provide care to patients who could not be treated adequately at primary (community hospital) or secondary (regional referral hospital) institutions. Tertiary-care hospitals are often affiliated with medical schools.

ACCP actively recruits members who practice clinical pharmacy in a variety of settings beyond the **tertiary-care institutions** where its early members worked. This has greatly increased its membership rolls and provided the group with increased political clout. ACCP was the driving force behind the recognition of pharmacotherapy as a certifiable pharmacy specialty in 1988 by the Board of Pharmaceutical (now Pharmacy) Specialties.

Currently, ACCP provides self-assessment programs, preparatory review courses, and recertification courses in various pharmaceutical specialties. Specifically, members have access to the Ambulatory Care Pharmacy Self-Assessment Program and Pharmacotherapy Self-Assessment Program; Critical Care, Pediatric, Oncology Preparatory Review Courses; and a Pharmacotherapy Recertification Course.[5]

ACCP conducts two conferences per year. An annual meeting, attracting more than 2,000 people, is conducted in late October or November; the conference is heavy on continuing education about clinical practice and research and includes little political activity (the college has no House of Delegates). A midyear research forum attracts several hundred attendees in April; it is popular among pharmacy residents preparing to take certification examinations.

The college has been very successful at establishing post-PharmD fellowships in advanced areas of pharmacotherapy (see Chapter 10). It is also an important part of the dialogue on recognition of pharmacists and direct patient care providers, the kinds of residencies and fellowships needed by pharmacy practitioners, and other issues on the interface between pharmacy education and clinical practice.

ACCP members are undoubtedly some of the best thinkers in pharmacy. They have led pharmacy to a point where society increasingly recognizes the value of the information and clinical management skills pharmacists offer patients. Their challenge today remains extending such services in such a way that all pharmacists—not just the best minds—can effectively provide them in a variety of types of pharmacy practice settings.

Academy of Managed Care Pharmacy

The Academy of Managed Care Pharmacy (AMCP) is one of pharmacy's newest and fastest-growing organizations. Founded in 1989, AMCP boasts 8,000 members and estimates that its members provide care to more than 200 million Americans served by managed care.

The academy conducts two meetings annually and publishes a newsletter and journal, *Journal of Managed Care Pharmacy*. Because of the rapid growth of managed care, attendance at AMCP meetings has swelled, and representatives of the pharmaceutical industry attend in large numbers to gain a better appreciation of this emerging market segment.

AMCP members strongly buy into the pharmaceutical care system. With members in health maintenance organizations, other types of managed care groups, and pharmacy benefit management companies, AMCP members are in a prime position to help define the appropriate roles for pharmacists in the years to come.

The rapid growth of managed care bodes well for AMCP. The importance of managed care pharmacy continues to increase as the positive influences of cost containment and quality of care are recognized and appreciated by an increasing number of health care payers.

Recently, the number of AMCP student pharmacists' chapters has been increasing. The purpose of the students' chapters is to educate future pharmacists on the expanding role of pharmacists in managed care. Given the rise of integrated health care systems and the Affordable Care Act, student pharmacists have opportunities in the growing fields of pharmacy administration, pharmacoeconomics, pharmaceutical marketing, and transitions of care.[6]

National Community Pharmacists Association

Founded in 1898 as the National Association of Retail Druggists, the National Community Pharmacists Association (NCPA) continues to build on its reputation for entrepreneurial programs that benefit community pharmacists and for championing community pharmacy on Capitol Hill. NCPA worked with industry partners to help build the fourth-largest Medicare Prescription Drug Program in the country, SilverScript, which was acquired by CVS in 2013. NCPA's members are entrepreneurs, and the association reflects those intrinsic characteristics.

NCPA is also well known and has been extremely active and effective in the governmental arena. It has been able to focus its lobbying efforts in Washington and at the state level, and the cohesiveness of its members can produce remarkably successful grassroots campaigns. And if there's one person a legislator does not want on the other side of an issue, it's the local pharmacist back home.

NCPA's members are based in the nation's 22,000-plus independent community pharmacies. As was noted in Chapter 6 on career paths, many of these pharmacies are anything but the standard corner drugstore—they often have multiple locations, offer intravenous admixture services, and boast long-term-care divisions that serve nursing homes. NCPA has historically been the organization of the pharmacy owners, but its memberships also includes pharmacy technicians and thousands of community staff pharmacists and pharmacy students.

NCPA conducts three meetings annually. The Annual Convention and Trade Exposition in October includes education, exhibits, and political activity in a House of Delegates. The Multiple Locations Pharmacy Conference, held during the winter in a location with a warm climate, is focused on continuing education, networking, and exhibits. Sites of these two meetings vary each year. The NCPA National Legislation and Government Affairs Conference, held in Washington, D.C., each May, attracts members who want to know more about and make a difference in the pharmacy-related laws and regulations being debated at the federal level.

NCPA publishes *America's Pharmacist* monthly, and it contains a wealth of information of use to the practicing community pharmacist. NCPA also publishes several newsletters, including some devoted to the home health and long-term-care fields. The *NCPA Digest* is an annual presentation of data and information about the professional and business aspects of community pharmacy practice.

NCPA responded aggressively to the advent of Medicare Part D and MTM. NCPA formed subsidiary organizations to both serve as a national provider of Medicare Part D services (now SilverScript) and partner with pharmacists to provide MTM services directly to patients (www.mirixa.com).

In 1991, NCPA expanded its commitment by launching a separate organization called the National Home Infusion Association (NHIA). NHIA is headquartered at NCPA and is devoted to legislative and regulatory representation, clinical continuing education, and management and marketing assistance for home infusion providers. NHIA holds an annual conference each year, and it publishes a bimonthly journal for its members, *Infusion*, as well as providing bulletins on emerging issues.

As reflected by its annual governmental conference, NCPA continues its long-standing commitment in this arena. It has been instrumental in gaining passage of several important pieces of legislation at both the federal and state levels. It was a key player in passage of federal pharmacy crime law, making robbery or burglary of a pharmacy a federal offense; the Prescription Drug Marketing Act, which combats illicit drug diversion; and the so-called Pryor legislation, requiring manufacturers to provide their best prices to Medicaid programs and pharmacists to offer patient counseling. In addition, the association is pursuing legislation regarding prompt payment for Medicare claims, tamper-resistant prescription pads for Medicaid prescriptions, and a fair reimbursement payment formula for Medicaid claims. The organization's efforts have led its political action committee to become one of the top 50 trade association political action committees in the country and to the formation of the Congressional Community Pharmacy Caucus to serve as a permanent platform for sharing ideas, news, and research on community pharmacy legislative issues on Capitol Hill.

NCPA has an aggressive student-outreach program that now features active student chapters in most of the nation's pharmacy schools. To attract more student pharmacists to community pharmacy, the association has developed information on community pharmacy ownership, including publications such as *Buying a Pharmacy: A "How-To" Guide*, a robust management section at www.ncpanet.org, and articles published in *America's Pharmacist* about young entrepreneurs who have been successful in independent practice and tips on how to get started in purchasing one's own pharmacy.

The mission of the chapters is to: "encourage, foster, and recognize an interest in community pharmacy ownership and entrepreneurship among the future leaders of their profession."[7] To empower student pharmacists to own their pharmacies, the NCPA and its foundation established the Good Neighbor Pharmacy NCPA Pruit-Schutte Student Business Plan Competition.[8] The main goal of this national competition is to promote entrepreneurship skills among future pharmacists. Many regional pharmacy associations have developed similar student business plan competitions for their annual meetings.

NCPA has successfully been able to shift the solutions it provides as times have changed community pharmacy. The organization continues to respond quickly and effectively as changes in pharmacy and health care present opportunities for its members, including students. The NCPA's National Student Leadership Council provides leadership, networking, and scholarship opportunities for student pharmacists.[9]

American Society of Consultant Pharmacists

Founded in 1969 by a group of entrepreneurs within pharmacy practice, the American Society of Consultant Pharmacists (ASCP) continues to reflect that spirit and drive. With a membership exceeding 9,000, the organization also has more than 5,700 student members. The society has no house of delegates; policy is developed by committees of members and approved by the board of directors.

ASCP members are experts in geriatric pharmacotherapy who treat medically complex and frail, elderly patients wherever they reside. As patient advocates, they are often known as "America's senior care pharmacists."

The ASCP's mission is as follows: "The American Society of Consultant Pharmacists empowers pharmacist and other healthcare professionals to enhance quality of care for all older persons through the appropriate use of medications and the promotion of healthy aging."[10] The ASCP's vision is "optimal medication management and improved health outcomes for all older persons."[10]

ASCP is fulfilling the dream of providing advanced pharmaceutical care to improve quality of life. ASCP members practice in a multitude of diverse settings. The majority of ASCP members practice in nursing facilities, followed by assisted living facilities and hospice care. Approximately one-third of the members practice in one of the following settings: acute care, hospital-based facilities, community pharmacy, or mental health facilities. Finally, one-third of the members practice in home settings and adult day care combined. Traditionally known for their federally mandated role in nursing facilities, ASCP members now are leading the way in delivering MTM and patient care services both under the Medicare Part D prescription drug benefit and in private-pay situations.

ASCP has two annual conventions, both of them a good mix of clinical, business, and regulatory educational sessions, balanced with exhibits and social networking functions. The ASCP Annual Meeting and Exhibition is held in October or November and attracts about 3,000 attendees. The ASCP Forum is held in the spring to provide members with an abbreviated-format conference. Both events offer continuing pharmacy education credit.

Information delivery through publications, including software and other new kinds of media, is an increasingly important service of ASCP. *The Consultant Pharmacist,* the society's Medline-indexed, peer-reviewed journal, mixes feature articles on current developments with practice-oriented research articles and departments. Its award-winning website, www.ascp.com, is rich with information. ASCP offers clinical references, practice development and regulatory and policy guides, and resources on business and management.

ASCP focuses heavily on building relationships with other pharmacy, aging, and long-term-care associations. ASCP holds a seat on the steering committee of PQA, a pharmacy quality alliance; its members and staff serve as co-chairs of the long-term-care quality metrics subcommittee.

ASCP also works closely with officials from the Centers for Medicare & Medicaid Services. It was ASCP that led the fight to protect the health and welfare of long-term-care residents, especially those who qualify for both Medicare and Medicaid ("dual-eligibles"), under the Medicare Modernization Act of 2005.

Given the growing number of older patients, ASCP provides continuing education programs to pharmacists and other geriatric health care professionals.[10] The ASCP's Professional Development Center has various learning activities to enhance members' competencies. Specifically, health care professionals will be able to "reflect, plan, act, and evaluate" their services to continuously enhance the quality of patient care.

American College of Apothecaries

The term *college,* when used in the name of a professional association, connotes more selective membership criteria or procedures than are used by *societies* or *associations*. So it is with the ACA. The ACA vision statement states: "Dedicated to the advancement of professional practice in independent community pharmacy through entrepreneurship and mentoring."[11] Its mission statement reads: "Dedicated to advancing the entrepreneurship spirit of member pharmacists through education, innovation, mentoring, fellowship, and training."[11]

Founded in 1940 by members of APhA, ACA has always represented the hopes and desires of pharmacists who wanted their colleagues to focus on the professional side of practice rather than on the business aspects. Thus, ACA members must meet certain criteria, including owning or working in a pharmacy that is devoid of commercialistic trappings or advertising. ACA pharmacies would fit in the category referred to as apothecary shops: those with limited or no "front-end" merchandise and that sell primarily prescription and nonprescription drugs, medical supplies, and related materials.

Today, ACA has full-time staff members at its offices in Memphis, Tennessee. It has two sister organizations, the ACA Research & Education Foundation, established in 1978, and the American College of Veterinary Pharmacists, founded in 1998. ACA's role in pharmacy politics has always been somewhat limited by its small membership and budget, but ACA members remain a very cohesive bunch.

ACA activities include the publication of several newsletters and two meetings annually, in the spring and autumn. ACA provides training courses, live webinars, and on-demand continuing education programs to its members.[11]

In many ways, ACA represents the professional aspirations of pharmacists who were dashed by the rush to commercialism and mass merchandising of the 1950s and 1960s. The same fuel that spurred the growth of outlets such as CVS, K-Mart, and Wal-Mart burned the hopes for universalization of a more professional level of pharmacy practice, one that required the half century described in Chapter 3 to re-emerge.

Pharmacy's alphabet soup

In addition to these major pharmacy practitioner organizations, several dozen other groups operate within pharmacy or on its periphery. Many of these are listed at the bottom of Table 8.1 or in Table 8.2. In addition, major pharmacy conventions and the general time frames when they usually occur are shown in Table 8.3.

Table 8.3 | Major Pharmacy Conventions

Sponsoring Organization	Convention
APhA–ASP	Midyear Regional Meetings/eight locations (see www.pharmacist.com)/Fall
APhA–ASP	APhA Annual Meeting/mid-March to early April
	Upcoming sites of APhA Annual Meeting: 2017, San Francisco; 2018, Nashville
NCPA	Annual Meeting/October
NCPA	NCPA Multiple Locations Conference/February
ACA	Annual Conference/October or November
ASHP	Midyear Clinical Meeting/early December
ASHP	Summer Meeting/June
ASCP	Annual Meeting/October or November
ASCP	ASCP Forum/April or May
ACCP	Annual Meeting/October to early November
ACCP	Spring Practice and Research Forum/April
NACDS	Pharmacy, Managed Care, and Technology Conference/late August
NACDS	Annual Meeting/late April
AMCP	Educational Conference/October
AMCP	Annual Meeting/April
NABP	Annual Meeting (see www.nabp.net)/May
NASPA	Meets at the APhA and NCPA annual meetings
AACP	Annual Meeting/July

For the student, the message is simple: get involved. To become a successful and contributing part of the profession of pharmacy, the student pharmacist must become integrated within the profession's patchwork of organizations. Through them, the student and young pharmacist can be nurtured professionally. Someday, the new practitioner can give back to the profession through involvement as a leader in one of these groups, so that pharmacy becomes even better. This is the expectation society has of a professional, and the professional association is the most common mechanism for actualizing that goal.

REFERENCES

1. JCPP Approves Pharmacists' Patient Care Process, June 14, 2014. American Pharmacists Association website. www.pharmacist.com/jcpp-approves-pharmacists-patient-care-process. Accessed April 19, 2016.

2. Accreditation Council for Pharmacy Education. *Accreditation Standards and Key Elements for the Professional Program in Pharmacy Leading to the Doctor of Pharmacy Degree ("Standards 2016").* Chicago: Accreditation Council for Pharmacy Education; 2015. www.acpe-accredit.org/deans/standardsrevision.asp. Accessed April 11, 2016.

3. APhA-ASP Midyear Regional Meetings (MRMs). American Pharmacists Association website. www.pharmacist.com/apha-asp-midyear-regional-meetings-mrms-0. Accessed April 11, 2016.

4. Student Societies. ASHP website. www.ashp.org/menu/MemberCenter/SectionsForums/PSF/Student-Societies.aspx. Accessed June 9, 2016.

5. American College of Clinical Pharmacy website. www.accp.com/about/mission.aspx. Accessed April 13, 2016.

6. Academy of Managed Care Pharmacy website. www.amcp.org. Accessed April 12, 2016.

7. NCPA Student Chapter Operations. NCPA website. www.ncpanet.org/students/chapter-operations. Accessed April 12, 2016.

8. Good Neighbor Pharmacy NCPA Pruit-Schutte Student Business Plan Competition. NCPA website. www.ncpanet.org/students/business-plan-competition. Accessed April 12, 2016.

9. NCPA National Student Council. NCPA website. www.ncpanet.org/students/leadership-opportunities. Accessed April 12, 2016.

10. About ASCP. American Society of Consultant Pharmacists website. www.ascp.com. Accessed April 13, 2016.

11. About ACA. American College of Apothecaries website. http://acainfo.org/about-aca/. Accessed April 12, 2016.

Chapter 9

Using the Pharmacy Literature— and Writing for It

L. Michael Posey

One characteristic of a profession is that it has its own body of literature. Thus, a corollary to this idea is that professionals should contribute to that literature. This chapter is included so that you can begin to envision your future role as a creator of knowledge about pharmacy and to inculcate in you the idea that pharmacy professionals always share new knowledge with colleagues for the benefit of all patients.

It is never too early to begin contributing to the pharmacy literature. As a student pharmacist or even prepharmacy student, you already are experiencing a part of the culture and traditions of pharmacy. As you do so, your thoughts and ideas about pharmacy or about pharmacy education could be of interest and value to the rest of the profession. A simple letter to the editor of a state or national publication could launch a noteworthy career as a pharmacist-author.

In this chapter, I describe the structure of the pharmacy literature, clues about ways of accessing it, and tips for contributing to it. Students who desire more information about pharmacy or biomedical literature should check their schools' curricula for courses in drug information or literature evaluation, or talk with pharmacy faculty members who publish frequently. In addition, talk with information specialists at your school or university library for help with literature searches and other resources.

Structure of the biomedical literature

Much of the scientific and biomedical literature, including that of pharmacy, is divided into three categories:

- Primary literature, such as original research articles, descriptive reports, case reports, opinions, and news articles
- Secondary literature, such as review articles that summarize the primary literature on a specific topic or abstracting/indexing services that provide information about where to look in the primary literature for specific types of information
- Tertiary literature, such as books and other major summaries of broad topics, including reference books

Most of this chapter is devoted to the primary literature. Pharmacy has numerous professional journals, news magazines, practice-oriented magazines, newsletters, and other regular periodicals (Table 9.1). Many industry-sponsored publications are available as well.

Among the components of the secondary pharmacy literature, foremost is International Pharmaceutical Abstracts (IPA). Created by the American Society of Health-System Pharmacists in 1964 and acquired by Thomson Scientific in 2005, IPA electronically provides

Table 9.1 | Selected Pharmacy Periodical Publications

Periodical Name/Address	Editor/Editor-in-Chief	Publisher/Website
Association newsletters and journals[a]		
Journal of the American Pharmacists Association	Andy Stergachis	APhA
Pharmacy Today	Kristin Weitzel	APhA
APhA DrugInfoLine	Randy C. Hatton	APhA
Journal of Pharmaceutical Sciences	Ronald T. Borchardt	APhA
Student Pharmacist	Tom English	APhA–ASP
America's Pharmacist	Michael F. Conlan	NCPA
NCPA Newsletter	Michael F. Conlan	NCPA
Infusion	Jeannie Counce	NHIA
Journal of Managed Care Pharmacy	Laura E. Happe	AMCP
AMCP News	Kevin Bruns	AMCP
American Journal of Health-System Pharmacy	Daniel J. Cobaugh	ASHP
ASHP Intersections	Kathleen Biesecker	ASHP
The Consultant Pharmacist	H. Edward Davidson	ASCP
ASCP Update	Marlene Bloom	ASCP
Pharmacotherapy	C. Lindsay DeVane	ACCP
ACCP Report	Kim Seiz	ACCP
American Journal of Pharmaceutical Education	Gayle A. Brazeau	AACP
Academic Pharmacy Now	Maureen Thielemans	AACP
Pharmaceutical Research	Peter Swaan	AAPS
Other publications		
Annals of Pharmacotherapy		aop.sagepub.com
ComputerTalk for the Pharmacist		www.computertalk.com
Drug Store News		www.drugstorenews.com
Drug Topics		drugtopics.modernmedicine.com
FDA Drug Safety Newsletter		www.fda.gov/Drugs/DrugSafety/DrugSafetyNewsletter/
FDC Reports ("The Pink Sheet")/Health News Daily		www.pharmamedtechbi.com/publications/the-pink-sheet; www.pharmamedtechbi.com/publications/health-news-daily
Hospital Pharmacy		archive.hospital-pharmacy.com
Journal of Pharmacy Practice		jpp.sagepub.com
Pharmacist's Letter		pharmacistsletter.therapeuticresearch.com
Pharmacy Times		www.pharmacytimes.com
U.S. Pharmacist		www.uspharmacist.com

[a] See Chapter 8 for association addresses and Web links (Table 8.1).

abstracts of pharmacy literature from around the world (https://health.ebsco.com/products/international-pharmaceutical-abstracts). It can be searched online through TOXLINE, a searchable **computerized database** available through several **database vendors** (including Cambridge Scientific Abstracts, DataStar, Dialog, DIMDI [German Institute of Medical Documentation and Information], EBSCO, Optionline div.PTI, Ovid, SilverPlatter, and STN) and many medical libraries.

In addition, most pharmacy journals regularly publish review articles about diseases, drugs, and other pharmacy topics. Some are devoted entirely to review and survey articles.

Two other key indexing services are very useful for pharmacists and student pharmacists. *Index Medicus* is the indexing publication of the National Library of Medicine, and it is available online as PubMed (www.pubmed.gov). *Index Medicus* includes much of the pharmacy literature and virtually all of the important medical literature; thus, it is the key source used for clinically oriented literature searches. The other publication, *Science Citation Index (SCI),* is a publication of the Institute of Scientific Information in Philadelphia. *SCI* lists previously published articles and all subsequent articles that have used the older article as a reference. Suppose, for example, that you are preparing a paper on heart transplants. You could look in *SCI* for one of the early articles from the 1960s on heart transplants and there find all later articles that cited the original works. *SCI* thus provides a valuable check on the accuracy of computerized literature searches and provides a way to come forward in the literature.

Pharmacy's tertiary literature is also very broad. Although entire libraries could be filled with these texts, a few key reference books are listed in Table 9.2.

With that background to the pharmacy literature as a whole, let's look at the process many authors go through when writing articles for publication. Although examples from the primary literature are used, the same steps and principles would apply to other kinds of professional writing, from patient newsletters to review articles for journals to chapters in books.

Writing for publication

When it comes right down to it, writing for publication is no different from writing in your diary. It's just that a lot more people will read it.

The biggest obstacle to writing—writer's block—is a psychological phenomenon that every writer in the world has experienced. The only real cure for it that I have found so far is a firm deadline, usually combined with pressure from an editor, publisher, coauthor, preceptor, or mentor. Because most pharmacists do not have such a person to keep them on track, we procrastinate and procrastinate and procrastinate. However, help is available—by forcing yourself to write, regardless of how painful it may seem. Write about anything, but make yourself express your thoughts through the written word. Don't worry about format or spelling or structure or organization—just write. A good editor can fix it later—the hard part is getting started.

Abstracts:
A short (100–200 words) summary of an article. Abstracts may merely describe the scope of an article, or they may present the key points or data presented in the paper.

Computerized databases:
Used in reference to the literature, this term means computer files containing information from articles that have been published in journals, magazines, and newspapers. These databases are searchable, using either key words from the title or abstract of the article, the authors' names, or the journals' names.

Database vendors:
Companies or organizations that obtain several databases and make them available to the public or others. Examples include BioMed Central, BIOSIS, CINAHL, MEDLINE with Full Text, and PubMed.

Table 9.2 | Key Pharmacy References

- *Remington: The Science and Practice of Pharmacy.* 22nd ed. Philadelphia: Pharmaceutical Press;2012.
- *Physicians' Desk Reference.* Oradell, N.J.: Medical Economics Co. Updated annually.
- *AHFS Drug Information.* Bethesda, Md.: American Society of Health-System Pharmacists. Updated annually.
- *Facts and Comparisons.* St. Louis, Mo.: Lippincott. Updated annually.
- *Handbook of Nonprescription Drugs: An Interactive Approach to Self-Care.* 18th ed. Washington, D.C.: American Pharmacists Association;2015. Updated every 3 years.
- Drugdex and Poisindex. Denver: Thomson/Micromedex. Updated annually.
- *Goodman and Gilman's The Pharmacological Basis of Therapeutics.* 12th ed. New York: McGraw-Hill;2011. Updated every 5 years.
- *Koda-Kimble and Young's Applied Therapeutics: The Clinical Use of Drugs.* 10th ed. Baltimore: Lippincott Williams & Wilkins;2012. Updated every 4 years.
- *Pharmacotherapy: A Pathophysiologic Approach.* 9th ed. New York: McGraw-Hill;2014. Updated every 3 years.

"Many pharmacists are good writers; to most of them, including the widely published stars, writing does not come naturally or easily. They sweat over their master-pieces, word after word, draft after crumpled draft. Although there are rare exceptions whose first drafts read with the grace and fluency of an E. B. White essay, most good writers have achieved this distinction through hard work. They have high standards and the perceptive-ness to recognize when their work is only half done."

—William A. Zellmer, in "How to Write a Research Report for Publication," *Research in Pharmacy Practice: Principles and Methods,* 1981:142

Of course, a common form of writer's block is provided by the tortuous process of deciding what to write about. Whereas authors of research projects have usually spelled out a great many parts of the final article at various stages of conducting the project, authors of opinion pieces or descriptive reports do not have this advantage. All I can say is this: if you can imagine that any other pharmacist in the country or even in the world might encounter the same problem or situation that you have and not know precisely how to handle it, then you have the kernel of some type of publication. In more than 30 years of editing pharmacy journals, I have seen reports published such as the one in which the primary original thought was to cut the top off a box of intravenous fluid bottles and use the resulting cubbyholes for sorting medication orders as they came from nursing units in a hospital. I have seen scientifically questionable articles published because they were timely, and I have seen seemingly irrelevant articles published because they were scientifically valid. Simply put, most articles in the professional literature are not earth-shaking pieces of research; some of the most valuable are simply practical tips on how a pharmacist solved an everyday problem.

Also remember that several different types of articles can be published. Research articles are subjected to rigorous scientific review, but many journals and magazines have sections for descriptive reports, letters to the editor, and editorials (Table 9.3). Think about what you want to say, and then look at the journal to which you want to submit your article. Write your article like those in the section where you think the content of your article will fit.

Once a topic is identified, the next step is to read related articles that have already been published. As a pharmacy resident, I wasted 2 or 3 months growing bacteria in intravenous and parenteral nutrition solutions only to find out that microbiology researchers had published the same studies nearly 10 years earlier. One rule that editors of pharmacy journals won't usually break is that articles should not reinvent the wheel.

In preparing for the day when you want to put your hands on the keyboard, consider these tips:
- Read books about writing well (as listed in Table 9.4).
- Regularly read publications that are well written and well edited. Emulate them. They are the best models available.
- Take courses in grammar, composition, or other skills that need improvement.

Table 9.3 | Types of Articles in the Pharmacy Literature

• Research paper	• Editorial
• Case report	• Book review
• Reviews and case-series analysis	• Letter to the editor

Note: For advice on how to write each type of paper, consult: Huth EJ. *Writing and Publishing in Medicine*. 3rd ed. Baltimore: Williams & Wilkins;1999.

- Purchase a good style manual (Table 9.4) appropriate for your writing needs. Read it for understanding, and study its preferences and principles. Write with the necessary tools at hand or available in your word-processing software, including a dictionary, thesaurus, and when appropriate, a medical dictionary and style manual.
- Always write for the specific journal and audience for which the article is intended.
- Have your writing critiqued by professors or colleagues whose skills are well developed. Heed their comments—criticism may be hard to take at first, but those comments that hit the hardest usually contain an element of truth.
- Write every time you can. Write reports for class; prepare articles for school organizations and publications; contribute to your pharmacy college newsletter and state pharmacy journal. Analyze the feedback you receive.
- Review the instructions for authors of the publication to which you plan to submit. If you cannot find them, contact the editor and request a copy. Read these closely before you begin writing.
- Develop a system for writing. Find a subject and make a list. Organize the list into an outline. Always write in an appropriate location or situation, or with a certain pen or color of paper, or with a certain word-processing program. Write when you are fresh, not tired or frustrated. Minimize distractions and interruptions.
- Write, rewrite, edit, and revise. There is one best way to express a thought. Find it.
- After a paper is perfect, have colleagues critique it. Then revise it again—cut out the fat, but leave the arteries intact. Every good writer needs an editor; use the feedback to improve accuracy and clarity of the article.

When writing an article, begin with the part of it that you find the easiest to put on paper. For instance, in a research article, the hardest part to write is often the introduction. Start with something very straightforward, such as the tables and figures or the methods. These parts involve less creativity, and they are the parts that you know best. They should be easy to put down on paper, and seeing the article begin to coalesce will give you the drive to keep going.

Table 9.4 | Tools for Improving Writing

Type	Publication
Dictionaries	• *American Heritage Dictionary*: Includes helpful style and usage notes
	• *Stedman's Medical Dictionary*, 27th ed.: Also available on disk with medical and pharmaceutical terms (including drug names) for use with many word-processing programs
Style manuals	• Council of Biology Editors, *CBE Style Manual*, 5th ed.: Very good for scientific papers
	• *AMA Manual of Style*, 10th ed.: The best guide for medical and clinical manuscripts
Writing style and grammar	• *The Elements of Style*, 3rd ed.: Also known as Strunk and White; a classic book on the philosophy of modern writing
	• *Writing and Publishing in Medicine*, 3rd ed.: An excellent discussion of how to prepare papers for biomedical journals and what happens to them after they are submitted

Note: These books are readily available in most college bookstores, especially those on medical campuses, and online at www.amazon.com and other online book vendors.

After the methods, tables, and figures are done, draft the results and discussion sections. The results flow logically from the methods, and the discussion should put your results in perspective with previously published material on the same or similar subjects.

Finally, at the end, draft the conclusion and introduction sections. The conclusion should flow logically from the study objectives that you set at the beginning of the project, and you can now write the perfect introduction to the paper. Finalize your references once the introduction is in place, and get ready to provide your first draft to some friends or colleagues who can give you critical feedback.

The revision process for a manuscript is designed to accomplish two goals: to improve your paper's accuracy (conveying what really happened or how the research was actually conducted) and your paper's clarity (saying what happened in such a way that people not involved in the project can understand). The best technique for accomplishing these goals is to have the first draft reviewed by other people who know the situation (review for accuracy, often performed by coauthors of the paper), incorporate those comments, and then have the paper reviewed by others not familiar with the manuscript (review for clarity). If the comments from these two rounds of review are minimal, the manuscript is ready for submission for publication.

Peer review in biomedical publishing

When the editor receives your manuscript for publication, he or she has two primary questions: Is the paper of interest to the readers of this journal, and is it accurate and clear in its presentation? To answer these questions, the advice of outside reviewers who are knowledgeable in your content area is often sought.

Peer review:
Analysis of submitted articles by experts who are not part of the journal's staff.

The process of obtaining this outside review is known in biomedical publishing as the **peer-review process.** For many pharmacy journals, the process is double-blinded: neither the reviewers nor the authors know the identity of the other party. Other journals use a partially blind system in which the authors are known to the reviewers, but the reviewers' identities are masked to the authors. A few journals use a fully open process in which both parties know the identity of the other. The editors have an ethical obligation to provide the author with the contents of the reviewers' critiques, regardless of whether the editor agreed with them, but the editor does not disclose the identity of the other parties without their express permission.

The editor usually arrives at one of four decisions about submitted manuscripts:
- Accept for publication.
- Revise before publication.
- Clarify before a decision can be reached.
- Reject.

In writing to the author, the editor clearly states one of these four options. Very few papers are accepted outright with no changes requested of the author. The second option creates a kind of legal contract between the editor and the author; the editor is saying that if the author will make or agree to certain changes in the paper, then the paper will be published. Letters expressing option 3 carry no such commitment; in particular, authors receiving a letter asking for clarification often find that the editor seeks again the advice of outside reviewers before reaching a decision.

If changes to an article are made as requested, the editor will normally accept the paper and schedule it for publication.

Copyediting and steps in the production process

Following acceptance of a paper for publication, the journal's staff will **copyedit** the paper to conform with the style of that periodical. Some authors are surprised at the extent of editing, but most agree that the changes improve the clarity and accuracy of the manuscript.

The **style manual** of a publication is used by the editors to create a familiarity with the content among regular readers. In short, the editor wants the journal to be as comfortable to readers as slipping on a pair of favorite shoes. For instance, a certain term may always be used when referring to a certain disease. Common abbreviations may not be spelled out on first mention. Editors may move parts of the paper around to what they consider a clearer or more logical flow of ideas. And, of course, overt spelling or grammatical errors are corrected.

Authors of major articles in pharmacy journals will receive one or more proofs of the article before it goes to print. Many journals today provide the edited manuscript as a word-processing file. These are usually followed by a set of page proofs that show the article as it will appear in the journal. At these stages, be certain to read the article very closely, and question changes that you feel have altered the meaning of the article. Good editing is like good surgery: it removes the fat but leaves the muscles and blood vessels intact. If the editors have massacred parts of your paper, then challenge them to defend their changes. If the only answer they can provide is, "It sounds better this way," or "That's just our style," then ask them to use your version. After all, your name is on the paper!

The editors see one or more proofs of the article after the first set of page proofs, and soon the journal will be mailed to pharmacists throughout the country and around the world. You will suddenly be famous, with some people viewing you as an expert on the subject. You will certainly want to let your professional colleagues as well as friends and family know that you've been published!

Sharing your ideas with colleagues: Your ticket to fame and fortune

Even if you never pen a phrase that is printed in the pharmacy literature, the odds are still 100% that you will be called on to write something during your pharmacy career. It may be an article for the local newspaper about a new drug, a proposal for providing services to a home health agency or nursing home, a memorandum for employees of a pharmacy, or simple instructions on how to administer a prescription. Whatever the time and place, the principles spelled out in this chapter will apply, and the quality of your written presentation will affect the response of the readers. Writing is simply a skill that all pharmacists must hone in today's practice environment.

Copyediting:
Correction and preparation of a manuscript for typesetting and printing.

Style manual:
A book listing preferred ways of stating material in a field or publication.

Chapter 10

Postgraduate Educational and Training Opportunities

Abir A. (Abby) Kahaleh

Although the end of pharmacy school may seem a lifetime away, now is the time to begin planning your postgraduate education. Even for the decreasing number of you who will graduate and enter practice immediately, your education cannot end then. Pharmacy school provides an excellent basis for entering practice, but there is more to learn after you graduate—much, much more.

Why do pharmacy graduates need residencies?

In a recent *Pharmacy Today* article, an author addressed a common question that you may be contemplating in the near future: "Why do we have residencies anyway?"[1] This important question has several answers.

First, pharmacy graduates gain basic knowledge and skills during their doctor of pharmacy (PharmD) programs. Given the limited time they have in pharmacy school, they are only able to apply their knowledge in "real-world" settings during experiential education. On average, experiential education totals about 2,000 hours. For pharmacy graduates to master their skills, they will need close to 10,000 hours of direct patient care to become competent independent practitioners.[1]

Second, given the complexity of today's health care system, most practice settings are focusing on meeting specific quality measures to enhance patient outcomes. Several studies illustrate the value of having pharmacy residents at institutions. For example, a survey of academic medical centers conducted among hospital administrators, directors of pharmacy, and residency preceptors revealed that almost all preceptors (90%) stated that having pharmacy residents reduced medication errors, improved prescribers' behaviors, and enhanced medication use.[2]

Likewise, another article indicated that having postgraduate clinical training for pharmacists is essential for saving patients' lives.[3] The authors state that the most common prescribing errors are giving the wrong doses and missing drug–drug interactions. Because of aging patient populations, existence of comorbidities, and increased complexity of medication regimens, the authors argue that expecting student pharmacists to practice independently immediately after graduation may not be realistic. They conclude their argument by supporting the American Society of Health-System Pharmacists' long-range vision for the pharmacy workforce in hospitals: "Pharmacists in focused, direct patient care roles should complete an accredited post-graduate year 1 pharmacy residency in a hospital or health system and, preferably, become board certified in a pharmaceutical specialty."[4]

Learning Objectives

Upon completion of this chapter, the reader should be able to:

1. Explain the rationale for postgraduate education.

2. Understand the advantages of completing a residency or fellowship program.

3. Identify resources for pursuing postgraduate education and training.

"The true value of a residency is that it provides you with an unparalleled opportunity to gain competence, confidence, and a competitive edge. There is no other choice that you could make for that first year out of school that would give you the same comprehensive results in so short a time.... The career-long value of the residency experience is irreplaceable. It more than offsets the short-term financial sacrifice that is required."

—David Vogel and Anne Blake
Why pursue a residency?
Am J Hosp Pharm. 1991; 48:1878.

Third, pharmacy graduates develop their leadership skills during residency programs. A publication on pharmacy residency linked clinical services to effective leadership skills.[5] The authors indicate that because pharmacists are the medication safety experts, their role requires having effective management and leadership skills to establish and successfully implement organizational improvements. Pharmacists play a critical role in managing finance, technology, formulary, supply chain, and human resources. Consequently, it is essential for pharmacy graduates to develop their leadership skills in addition to their clinical skills for them to become effective medication safety experts.

Finally, from an economic perspective, completing a residency is beneficial to pharmacy graduates and institutions. A study examined the return on investment of having pharmacy residents at a Veterans Affairs hospital.[6] The residents' productivity was measured by "notations in progress notes" and compared with their pharmacist preceptors. The benefit-to-cost ratio of the residency program was higher than the ratio of hiring new, nonresidency-trained pharmacists. Another study evaluated the economic and clinical impact of a pharmacy resident at a large academic medical center.[7] The researchers compared the cost savings and cost avoidance for interventions made by the pharmacy resident with the costs and benefits of the residency program, confirming a net benefit of $55,821 during the 4-month study period.[7] The pharmacy resident also provided pharmaceutical care services and in-service educational programs to other professionals at the academic medical center. Furthermore, the physicians indicated that having a pharmacy resident on rounds was beneficial because they optimize medication use.

The purpose of this chapter is to stimulate you to begin exploring the various postgraduate opportunities that are available. Among the formal educational options open to the new pharmacy graduate are residencies, fellowships, traineeships, and graduate school. Let's look at what each of these entails.

Residency:
A postgraduate program of organized training that meets the requirements of a residency-accreditation body.

Residencies

Student pharmacists are increasingly choosing to go into **residency** programs after graduation. This path may soon be just as common for a pharmacist as it has been for physicians.

Residencies are valuable experiences because they offer a systematic educational focus in a real-world setting using a Socratic method of teaching. Each residency program is led by a preceptor who takes personal responsibility for ensuring that each resident has a quality learning experience. Through rotations in various clinical or other areas, pharmacy residents have the opportunity to learn about different types of patients and how various parts of the pharmacy or facility work by talking directly with patients, physicians, nurses, and pharmacy managers or supervisors. Although these skills and this knowledge may be gained in other ways, the residency facilitates acquisition in a short time.[8,9]

Pharmacy residency programs are now available in the areas shown in Table 10.1. Sources of current information about residency programs are the ASHP (www.ashp.org) and American Pharmacists Association (APhA) websites (www.pharmacist.com). A comprehensive list of available residencies and fellowships is maintained on the American College of Clinical Pharmacy (ACCP) website (www.accp.com).

Residencies have been common in hospital and health-system pharmacy since the 1960s, and they are now spreading to community pharmacies. First begun in the mid-1980s, community pharmacy residencies have grown in prominence and number since the late 1990s. Numerous community pharmacy residency programs are now accredited, and they offer a growing number of slots for innovative student pharmacists who want to expand medication therapy management into the nation's chain and independent community pharmacies.[10-14]

In 2003, ASHP reorganized its accreditation standards into a postgraduate year 1 (PGY1) and year 2 (PGY2). PGY1 programs can be conducted at one or more sites, and colleges of pharmacy can participate as sponsoring organizations. Residents learn about managing and improving the medication-use process, providing evidence-based, patient-centered medication therapy management with interdisciplinary teams, exercising leadership and practice management skills, demonstrating project management skills, providing medication and practice-related education and training, and using medical informatics.

PGY2 pharmacy residency programs focus on a specific area of practice, such as primary care/ambulatory, critical care, drug information, geriatrics, oncology, psychiatric, internal medicine, and other areas listed in Table 10.1.

Table 10.1 | Types of Pharmacy Residency Programs

Year	Program Type
Postgraduate year 1 residencies	• Community pharmacy
	• Managed care pharmacy
	• Pharmacy
Postgraduate year 2 residencies	• Ambulatory care pharmacy
	• Cardiology pharmacy
	• Critical care pharmacy
	• Drug information
	• Emergency medicine pharmacy
	• Geriatric pharmacy
	• Health-system pharmacy administration
	• Infectious disease pharmacy
	• Informatics
	• Internal medicine pharmacy
	• Managed care pharmacy systems
	• Medication-use safety
	• Nuclear pharmacy
	• Nutrition support pharmacy
	• Oncology pharmacy
	• Pediatric pharmacy
	• Pharmacotherapy
	• Psychiatric pharmacy
	• Solid organ transplant pharmacy

ASHP uses a resident-matching program in which both programs and applicants submit lists of their preferences; programs are then matched with their selected applicants who rank them the highest. Because of this national program, the deadlines for making application are not flexible, and interviews must be completed so that a program will be able to rank each person adequately before the deadline for submission of rankings.

Stipends for residencies are generally about one-half of what a starting pharmacist would earn. Benefits of employment are usually provided.

Other kinds of residencies are also available; these were mentioned in Chapter 6 in the discussion of alternative career paths in industry, government, and associations. Yearlong residencies are also available to student pharmacists after graduation. Contact the organizations at the addresses shown in Table 8.1 for more information.

Fellowships and traineeships

Fellowship:
A postgraduate program, usually research-oriented, often in a narrow field of study that relies on a Socratic teaching method.

Socratic teaching method:
The transfer of knowledge that relies on a person teaching one or a few students in a highly individualized manner. Named after Socrates of ancient Greece.

Traineeship:
Short-term programs, usually of one week in duration, that provide intensive information and demonstrations about one disease or a small group of similar conditions.

The important distinction between a residency and a **fellowship** is that the residency is practice-oriented whereas the fellowship has a research focus. In addition, where one preceptor might have several residents in a given pharmacy training, there is usually only one fellow, thereby increasing opportunity for the **Socratic style of teaching**. In recent years, **traineeships** have grown in number and popularity as practicing pharmacists have sought ways to enhance their knowledge and skills without interrupting their practices for an extended (usually one-year) residency or fellowship.

Many different areas—most of them clinical—are now available for pharmacists interested in completing a fellowship (Table 10.2). The major sponsor of fellowships is the ACCP Research Institute. It uses grants from the pharmaceutical industry to support the fellowship programs. Typically, the fellowships are not conducted at the sponsoring companies; hospitals and institutions apply for funding and then select an individual for the fellowship.

As with residencies, stipends for fellowships are about one-half of a starting pharmacist's salary. Employment benefits are usually provided. Fellowships, which may last for one or two years, are intensive research-oriented experiences and are therefore excellent ways to prepare for a career in academia or pharmaceutical industry. The fellow generally spends the entire time on a small number of research projects, including formulating the methods, conducting the research, and writing a manuscript for publication.

Traineeships are generally conducted for a few days (often from Sunday through Friday) at leading institutions or facilities specializing in the disease or area of interest. A limited number of pharmacists are accepted for each session, and they learn the latest concepts in clinical areas such as those listed in Table 10.2.

Using this intensive experience as a springboard, the practitioners then take their new skills and knowledge back to their practice setting, where they implement what they have learned in the traineeships. In some cases, pharmacists continue their training through interactions with local groups with interests in that disease or condition.

Table 10.2 | Available Fellowships and Sponsoring Organizations

Funding Sponsor	Type of Fellowship or Traineeship
ASHP Research and Education Foundation (www.ashpfoundation.org/ MainMenuCategories/Traineeships)	Antithrombotic Pharmacotherapy Traineeship Critical Care Traineeship Medical Home Traineeship Oncology Patient Care Traineeship Pain and Palliative Care Traineeship
American College of Clinical Pharmacy Research Institute	Access the ACCP Directory of Residencies, Fellowships, and Graduate Programs at www.accp.com/resandfel/
American Society of Consultant Pharmacists Research and Education Foundation (http://ascpfoundation.org/traineeships/index.cfm)	Parkinson's Disease Pharmacotherapy Traineeship

Graduate studies

For the student who wishes to pursue a research-oriented career in academia or pharmaceutical industry, graduate school is often the best path. Graduate studies are academically based experiences that focus on the student's research abilities, including literature review and analysis, statistical expertise, communication skills, and in-depth knowledge of the field of study.

The lack of students entering graduate studies—especially American-born student pharmacists—has been a concern of some in the profession. The concern relates to the fact that most pharmacy school faculty are products of such graduate work, and without pharmacists who have completed master's or doctor of philosophy degrees to mix with the nonpharmacists in those positions, the coursework offered may become less relevant to practice. Various techniques for increasing the interest of student pharmacists in graduate work have been proposed and tested.[15]

Many strong graduate programs are available in pharmacy and related disciplines. Lists and contract information for graduate programs at U.S. colleges of pharmacy are available on the American Association of Colleges of Pharmacy website (www.aacp.org/ resources/student/Pages/default.aspx).

In addition to the graduate pharmacy courses listed, many pharmacists have chosen to enter business, law, or medical schools. Depending on your overall career objectives, you may wish to consult with a career-counseling office at your school or university for more information about such options.

To apply to most graduate schools, you will need to take the Graduate Record Examination or other national tests and provide the school with transcripts and references. The graduate school to which you plan to apply can provide information about these items.

Pharmacy education: A lifelong learner

As was noted at the beginning of this book, change is a constant part of today's pharmacy world. Not only does pharmacy school *not* teach its students everything they need to know for pharmacy practice, but the amount of information known by the human race is now doubling every few years. No one—in any field—can leave school and assume that they know everything they will need to be a good practitioner for a lifetime. There are always new drugs, new diseases, new ideas, and new laws. The learning really never stops, and the potential opportunities offered by residencies, fellowships, traineeships, and graduate school should be seriously considered by every pharmacy graduate as a means of being well prepared to deal with the pharmacy world of today and tomorrow.

REFERENCES

1. McDonough RP. Why do we need residencies? *Pharm Today*. 2016;22(4):38.
2. Fuller PD, Smith KM, Hinman RK, et al. Value of pharmacy residency training: a survey of the academic medical center perspective. *Am J Health-Syst Pharm*. 2012;69(2):158–65.
3. Ibrahim RB, Ibrahim LB, Reeves D. Mandatory pharmacy residencies: one way to reduce medication errors. *Am J Health-Syst Pharm*. 2010;67(6):477–81.
4. American Society of Health-System Pharmacists. ASHP long-range vision for the pharmacy workforce in hospitals and health systems. *Am J Health-Syst Pharm*. 2007;64:1320–30.
5. Ivey MF, Farber MS. Pharmacy residency training and pharmacy leadership: an important relationship. *Am J Health-Syst Pharm*. 2011;68:73–76.
6. Pasek PA, Stephens C. Return on investment of a pharmacy residency training program. *Am J Health-Syst Pharm*. 2010;67(22):1952–7.
7. Daghstani A, Patel N. Economic and clinical impact of a pharmacy resident at a large academic medical center. *Hosp Pharm*. 2012;47(3):214–8.
8. Vogel D, Blake A. Why pursue a residency? *Am J Hosp Pharm*. 1991;48(9):1878.
9. Miller WA. Postgraduate residency education and training: a call for action. *Am J Pharm Educ*. 1989;53(3):310–1.
10. Posey LM. Rachel Henderson: ensuring pharmacy's role in MTM. *Pharm Today*. 2006;12(9):20–4.
11. Egervary A. Pharmacy professor and Rite Aid collaborate on community MTM. *Pharm Today*. 2007;14(9):36–9.
12. Pruchnicki MC, Rodis JL, Beatty SJ, et al. Practice-based research network as a research training model for community/ambulatory pharmacy residents. *J Am Pharm Assoc*. 2008;48(2):191–202.
13. Unterwagner WL, Zeolla MM, Burns AL. Training experiences of current and former community pharmacy residents, 1986–2000. *J Am Pharm Assoc*. 2003;43(2):201–6.
14. Rupp MT. Program planning for a community pharmacy residency support service using the nominal group technique. *J Am Pharm Assoc*. 2002;42(4):646–51.
15. Draugalis J, Bootman JL, McGhan WF, Larson LN. Attitudes of pharmacy students toward graduate education and research activities: suggestions for recruitment activities. *Am J Pharm Educ*. 1989;53:111–20.

Glossary

Abstracts:

A short (100–200 words) summary of an article. Abstracts may merely describe the scope of an article, or they may present the key points or data presented in the paper.

Accreditation:

Recognition of a residency or other type of program by comparing it with standards set by the accrediting body. This standard describes the goals or ideals that each program should strive for and sets certain minimum criteria that each should maintain.

Adherence:

The rate at which patients actually take a prescribed treatment. Known formerly as compliance. A related term, persistence, describes the rate at which patients continue to take their medications over time.

Adulterated:

Products that have been changed or contaminated with impure or foreign substances.

Biopharmaceutics:

The study of a drug's physical and chemical properties as they relate to the effects of the drug on the body (absorption, distribution, and metabolism or elimination).

Chronic conditions:

Diseases that last for more than about 6 months or that have long-term (usually lifelong) effects are referred to as chronic conditions. These include diabetes, hypertension (high blood pressure), and heart conditions. In addition, surgery and other therapies may produce a chronic condition. For instance, a colon cancer patient may have all or some of the colon removed, with an ostomy created for the passage of waste. Or a patient whose stomach is removed because of gastric cancer may require special types of enteral nutrition rather than a normal diet of solid foods.

Certification:

Recognition of an individual for specialized knowledge or skills based on demonstration of that knowledge or those skills to the certifying body. The term certification carries the connotation that the certifying body is a nongovernment entity, and the recognition typically carries no legally defined privileges.

Class of trade:

Customers of a business or industry may be divided into one or more groups based on their purchasing and payment characteristics. Each of these classes of trade is dealt with differently—and may receive different prices or payment policies—because of the interplay between these characteristics and the seller's goals and objectives relative to that part of the industry.

Closed-shop pharmacies:

A pharmacy not open to the public. It usually provides services to nursing homes or other types of long-term-care facilities. These services may be drug dispensing, consulting on patients' drug therapy, or both.

Code blue:

The hospital's response when a patient is in cardiopulmonary arrest (the heart and/or lungs have stopped). Various health care professionals respond to the code blue, and the pharmacist attends to help calculate doses and draw up drugs to be administered in this emergency situation. Hospitals differ in what they call the situation; code blue is a common term derived from the fact that the patient is turning blue from a lack of oxygen. Other names are code red or code 99.

Compounding:

The preparation of prescriptions specifically for a patient based on an individualized drug order from a prescriber.

Computerized databases:

Used in reference to the literature, this term means computer files containing information from articles that have been published in journals, magazines, and newspapers. These databases are searchable, using either key words from the title or abstract of the article, the authors' names, or the journals' names.

Controlled substances:

Any of several dangerous drugs, such as morphine, cocaine, codeine, diazepam (Valium), and amphetamines, that are handled, dispensed, and recorded specially under federal law.

Co-payment:

The amount of money a patient must pay when receiving certain types of health care services under insurance programs or prepaid health care plans.

Glossary

Copyediting:
Correction and preparation of a manuscript for typesetting and printing.

Covenant:
A promise or an agreement between two parties in which each provides something of value to the other. In pharmacy, the patient gives money to the pharmacist, who provides a patient-specific pharmaceutical product along with information on the proper use and adverse effects of that product.

Database vendors:
Companies or organizations that obtain several databases and make them available to the public or others. Examples include BioMed Central, BIOSIS, CINAHL, MEDLINE with Full Text, and PubMed.

Decentralized drug distribution:
Systems in hospitals of distributing drugs to patients in which pharmacy services are located in several locations near patient care areas rather than in one central pharmacy.

Deep discounter:
A type of mercantile outlet that reduces prices far below those of normal retail outlets and relies on volume to make a profit.

Drug information:
A service provided by pharmacists to other health professionals or to the public in which basic or detailed information about drugs is provided.

Drug interactions:
Detrimental (or occasionally positive) effects produced when two or more drugs are used at the same time. By checking the patient profile for interacting drugs, the computer can alert the pharmacist to consider whether both drugs can be safely used together in a patient.

Drug-regimen review:
A clinical pharmacy service provided to residents of nursing homes in which pharmacists review the drug therapy of residents and provide suggestions to physicians about drug selection, duplication, necessity, adverse effects, or monitoring.

Durable medical equipment:
Items such as wheelchairs, walkers, and bedside toilets that patients buy when their health fails or rent during rehabilitative periods after surgery or injury. The term can also include various types of intravenous (also called parenteral) or enteral services that require special catheters or pumps to safely deliver fluids or nutrition through the patient's veins or the gastrointestinal tract.

Efficacy:
The ability of a drug to produce desired therapeutic effects.

Emergency contraceptive:
Also known as the morning-after pill. Medication containing female hormones to be taken within 72 hours of unprotected intercourse that will prevent pregnancy more than 90% of the time.

Fellowship:
A postgraduate program, usually research oriented, often in a narrow field of study that relies on a Socratic teaching method.

Formulary:
A list of drugs that have been selected by the medical staff of a hospital or HMO for use in that institution. Drugs are selected on the basis of efficacy, safety, cost, and quality of life. In recent years, the marketing of many "me-too" drugs by the pharmaceutical industry—drugs that have no important advantage over drugs already on the market—has made cost an increasingly important factor in formulary decisions. Another important factor is the number of times per day that a medicine must be given, since in hospitals, highly paid personnel must dispense and administer each dose and in HMOs patient compliance is higher with fewer doses.

Galenicals:
Historically used to refer to a class of pharmaceutical products that were compounded through mechanical means.

Health care team:
A group of professionals with various skills who work together in providing patient care.

Hypochondriac:
A patient with a psychological disorder in which he or she complains of imagined medical problems.

Indigent:
Unable to pay for certain basic services for oneself, including health care.

Laws:
Acts passed by a legislative body.

License:
A document issued to pharmacists and other citizens that provides special privileges based on specialized knowledge or skills. A driver's license is one type of such document; it permits the holder to operate motorized vehicles on public roads based on a demonstration to the state of sufficient knowledge. A pharmacy license permits the holder to engage in a specialized profession known as pharmacy following demonstration to the state of adequate knowledge. It is a privilege, not a right, and thus the state may withdraw the privilege for various reasons.

Living will:
A legal document that provides guidance to health care professionals about what actions a patient would like taken if he or she is unable to provide an informed decision because of illness or injury. Also known as an advance directive.

Misbranded:
Drug products that are not properly labeled as to contents and proper use.

Negligence:
Failure of a professional to provide the standard of due care to patients who seek that care.

Nursing homes:
Facilities that provide residential care and health care to residents who live in them. Residents are typically deficient in one or more activities of daily living: ambulating, feeding, bathing, or toileting.

Nutrition support:
For patients whose medical conditions do not permit them to take a normal diet, nutrition support is provided. This may entail oral feedings using liquid foods or intravenous feedings using specialized solutions. The pharmacist is an important member of the nutrition support team because of special expertise in both product preparation and clinical areas.

Objectification:
The viewing of other people in a self-centered way, such as obstacles to one's own goals or a vehicle through which one's own goals can be realized without regard for the feelings of the other person.

Paradigm:
As used in this book, the typical or standard activities of a pharmacist on a day-to-day basis.

Patient carts:
Hospital pharmacies often use carts with small drawers, one for each patient on a nursing station, to deliver medications from a central or decentral pharmacy to the patient care floors. Each nursing-station cart is exchanged periodically, usually once a day, with a new supply of medications for each patient.

Patient profiles:
A record, usually computerized, of all medications a patient has received at a given pharmacy. Ideally, the profiles should include both prescription and nonprescription medicines.

Peer review:
Analysis of submitted articles by experts who are not part of the journal's staff.

Pharmacokinetic monitoring:
A part of pharmaceutical care required by patients on certain medications. For some drugs, the difference between a therapeutic blood level and a toxic blood level is very small, and the doses of those drugs need to be calculated carefully and blood levels checked to ensure optimal therapy.

Pharmacology:
The study of the action of drugs in biological systems.

Pharmacopeia:
Books listing drugs and other medical devices, including standards for their preparation and analysis, that are recognized by a governmental authority.

Pharmacy benefits managers (PBMs):
Companies that contract with managed care organizations, insurance companies, or employers to provide prescriptions and pharmaceutical care to a covered population. PBMs often contract with networks of independent or chain pharmacies to provide this care in accordance with guidelines and rules that can reduce the cost of prescriptions.

Pharmacy technician:
A paraprofessional assistant to the pharmacist who helps with the mechanical preparation of medications for dispensing to patients. This person may interpret prescription orders, prepare the medication (including some compounding of medications and preparation of intravenous solutions), and check the work of other technicians in specific situations.

Placebo:
A preparation with no known pharmacologic or medicinal properties. Placebos can sometimes "work" by making the patient believe that a real drug is being given, and placebos are used in some research as a way of identifying the beneficial properties of drugs.

Product labeling:
The information provided with a prescription drug, including the package insert that lists uses, precautions, adverse effects, and dosages of the drug product. The language used in the product labeling must be approved by FDA.

Reciprocation:
Once a pharmacist is licensed, he or she can use that license (if in good standing) to practice in other states, after the board of pharmacy in the new state recognizes the license from the previous state.

Regulations:
Rules promulgated by a part of the executive branch of government, usually based on a law giving the agency statutory authority for the regulation.

Residency:
A postgraduate program of organized training that meets the requirements of a residency-accreditation body.

Rounding:
Once or more often each day in a teaching hospital, members of the health care team gather to conduct "rounds", which usually involve walking to the room of each patient that team is currently caring for. Each member of the team has an opportunity to share with the others important information about the patient. Rounds also serve an important role in imparting knowledge among the members of the team.

Safety:
The ability of a drug not to produce harmful or deleterious side effects or adverse reactions.

Socratic teaching method:
The transfer of knowledge that relies on a person teaching one or a few students in a highly individualized manner. Named after Socrates of ancient Greece.

Glossary

Style manual:
A book listing preferred ways of stating material in a field or publication.

Terminal position:
A position in a corporate hierarchy from which one has little hope for advancement because of an individual's education and corporate policies.

Tertiary-care institutions:
Hospitals that provide care to patients who could not be treated adequately at primary (community hospital) or secondary (regional referral hospital) institutions. Tertiary-care hospitals are often affiliated with medical schools.

Traineeship:
Short-term programs, usually of one week in duration, that provide intensive information and demonstrations about one disease or a small group of similar conditions.

Unit dose packages:
In hospitals and some nursing homes, medications are packaged in strips, with each dose labeled with the brand name, strength, and generic name of the drug. Even though this packaging costs more, it speeds the pharmacy operation and permits return of unused medication to the pharmacy.

Wholesale druggists:
Intermediaries in the mercantile chain between manufacturers and retail outlets such as pharmacies.

Index

Page numbers followed by *t* and *f* indicate tables and figures, respectively.

Index

Index

G

galenicals 10
general stores 13
geriatric pharmacotherapy 99
Good Neighbor Pharmacy NCPA Pruit-Schutte Student
        Business Plan Competition 99
Gottlieb, J. 54
government
    careers in 75
    federal 29, 79-84
    internships 75
    programs (*See* Medicaid; Medicare)
    state 84-85
graduate studies 115
The Great American Fraud (Adams) 80
Griffenhagen, George 9

H

Handbook of Nonprescription Drugs 93
Healthcare Distribution Management Association 91*t*
Health Care Financing Administration 79, 82-84
health care team 67
health insurance 52-53
health maintenance claims 81
health maintenance organizations (HMOs) 72-74
Healthy People initiative 4
Helfland, William H. 9
Hepler, Charles D. 22, 26
heroic measures 50-51
Hilton Head conference (1985) 26
Hippocrates of Cos 10
Hippocratic Oath 46, 50
history of pharmacy 9-19
    ancient times 9-10, 10*t*, 21
    eighteenth century 13, 14*t*, 21
    Middle Ages 11, 11*t*, 21
    nineteenth century 15-17, 16*t*-17*t*, 22
    Renaissance 12*t*, 13
    twentieth century 17-19, 18*t*, 22, 23*t*-24*t*
HMOs (health maintenance organizations) 72-74
home care pharmacy 72-74
homeopathy 13
hospital pharmacy. *See* institutional pharmacy
Humphrey, Hubert H. 75
hypochondriac 45

I

iatrochemistry 13
Ibn Sina 11
illicit drugs 82
immediate language 42
immunizations 66-67
independent community pharmacies 62-64

indexing services 104-105
Index Medicus 104-105
Indian Health Service 75
indigent 83
infectious diseases 87
information
    disclosure of 49
    drug (*See* drug information)
informed consent 48-49
Infusion 98
Institute of Medicine (IOM) 31-32
Institute of Scientific Information 105
institutional pharmacy
    association (*See* American Society of Health-System
        Pharmacists)
    careers in 67-70
    decentralized drug distribution 25
    residencies in 86, 111, 113
International Pharmaceutical Abstracts (IPA) 103-104
International Pharmaceutical Federation (FIP) 91*t*
internships 59-60, 60*t*, 75-76, 86
interprofessional communication 40-42
interprofessional education 32
Interprofessional Education Collaborative (IPEC) 32
IPA (International Pharmaceutical Abstracts) 103-104
IPEC (Interprofessional Education Collaborative) 32

J

JCPP (Joint Commission of Pharmacy Practitioners) 89, 90*t*
Joint Commission of Pharmacy Practitioners (JCPP) 89, 90*t*
journals. *See* pharmacy literature; *specific publication*
Journal of the American Pharmacists Association 92
Journal of Managed Care Pharmacy 96
Journal of Pharmaceutical Sciences 92
The Jungle (Sinclair) 80
justice 46-48, 52-53

K

Kefauver-Harris Drug Amendments 80
killing, avoiding 46, 50-51

L

Lambda Kappa Sigma 60
Larsen, Magali Sarfatti 22
laws. *See also specific law*
    defined 79
    federal 29, 79-84
    state 84-85
leadership 75, 112
libertarianism 53
licenses 85
listening 37*f*, 37-38

Index

self-governance 85–87
state government 84–85
over-the-counter (OTC) medications 80–82

P

paintings (Robert Thom series) 9
paradigm 2
Parcelsus 13
Parker, Paul F. 24
paternalism 51–52
Pathways Evaluation Program for Pharmacy Professionals 57–59, 58f
patients
    autonomy of 46–49, 51–52
    competence of 48
    complaints by 37
    medication-taking behavior 36–39
patient adherence 38–39
patient care services. *See also* medication therapy management
    associations promoting 93
    in community pharmacies 63
    defined 31
    Pharmacists' Patient Care Process (JCPP) 89
    in public health 31–32
patient carts 68–69
patient-centered medical home (PCMH) 3
patient counseling. *See also* medication therapy management
    checklist for 41t
    communication during 39–40, 41t
    defined 40
    in Medicaid 2, 29
patient-pharmacist relationship
    communication in (*See* communications)
    covenant 28, 45
    development of 35–37
patient profiles 63
Patient Protection and Affordable Care Act 2, 79, 82–83
PBMs (pharmacy benefits managers) 5
PCMA (Pharmaceutical Care Management Association) 91t
PCMH (patient-centered medical home) 3
PCP (Philadelphia College of Pharmacy) 15
PDPs (prescription drug providers) 83
Peck, M.S. 36
pediatric pharmacy 87, 96
peer review 108–109
penicillin 19
Pen T'sao 9
people skills 61. *See also* communications
pharmaceutical care
    in community pharmacies 30–31
    core elements of 31
    defined 28t, 28–29
    in health systems 30–31

patient care (*See* patient care services)
    reprofessionalization and 22–29
Pharmaceutical Care Management Association (PCMA) 91t
pharmaceutical industry
    careers in 74–75
    history of 15, 17–19, 23
    internships 75
    pricing structure 84
Pharmaceutical Research and Manufacturers of America (PhRMA) 91t
pharmacists
    certification of 85–87, 93
    patient relationship with (*See* patient-pharmacist relationship)
    provider status 55, 79, 93
    role of 1–6, 24–33, 56
Pharmacists for the Future: The Report of the Study Commission on Pharmacy 26, 27t
Pharmacists' Patient Care Process (JCPP) 89
Pharmacists' Patient Care Services Digest (APhA) 31
pharmacokinetic monitoring 68
pharmacology 25
pharmacopeia 15
Pharmacopeia of the United States 15
pharmacotherapy 26, 87, 96
Pharmacotherapy 26, 96
Pharmacotherapy: A Pathophysiologic Approach 26
pharmacy
    history of (*See* history of pharmacy)
    oversight (*See* oversight)
    practice areas 61–62, 76, 77t
    as profession 17–19, 21–25
    self-governance by 85–87
    specialities in 86–87, 96
pharmacy associations 89–101. *See also specific association*
    versus boards of pharmacy 84–85
    chain pharmacists in 65–66
    conventions 101, 101t
    history of 13, 15
    internships 61, 76
    list of 91t
    management of 75–76
Pharmacy-Based Immunization Delivery certification program 66–67
pharmacy benefits managers (PBMs) 5
pharmacy education 111–116
    accreditation of 29, 85–86, 113–114
    entry-level degree 29
    fellowships 96, 114, 115t
    fraternities 60
    graduate studies 115
    history of 17, 19, 29
    internships 59–60, 60t, 75–76, 86
    interprofessional 31–32
    as lifelong experience 116
    pharmacy technicians 33, 86